Opportunities for Discovery

OPPORTUNITIES FOR DISCOVERY

Seeing What Others Do Not See

Martin G. Myers, MD, FRCPC
Division of Cardiology, Sunnybrook Health Sciences Centre
Professor Emeritus, Department of Medicine
University of Toronto

Rock's Mills Press
Rock's Mills, Ontario • Oakville, Ontario
2024

Published by
Rock's Mills Press
www.rocksmillspress.com

DEDICATION

I would like to acknowledge the contribution of my colleagues who collaborated on the studies mentioned in this book.

Contents

Introduction

Stella is a 64-year-old woman who has recently developed frequent headaches. Although she has been under considerable stress due to her husband's deteriorating health, she is still concerned that there may be something new happening. She decides it is time for a visit to her family doctor.

After her doctor listened to her story, she began the examination by recording Stella's blood pressure. The initial reading was 155/80 mmHg. She repeated the measurement and it was a little higher. Otherwise, Stella's story of her headaches was consistent with the increased stress she has been experiencing. Nothing else of importance was noted. Stella was told that her blood pressure was a little high and that she should return in two weeks to have it checked again. Not surprisingly, Stella became somewhat anxious about her high blood pressure.

Two weeks later, Stella was back in her family doctor's examining room for repeat blood pressure readings. The average of measurements was 152/82 mmHg, which Stella now recognizes to be higher than normal. Her family doctor decided it was time for medication, hoping to lower her blood pressure to normal.

Was the doctor's decision correct?

George is a 48-year-old salesman at a multinational company who travels frequently as part of his job. For years, he has drunk several cups of coffee at breakfast and one or two more later in the day. One day he read an article in the morning paper which said that drinking more than three cups of coffee a day could be associated with an increased risk of having a heart attack. George enjoyed his coffee and was under the impression that it improved his performance at work. He searched the internet for more information on coffee and heart disease and found several other studies which also suggested a link. Being very conscious about his health, George decided to switch to decaffeinated coffee.

Was his decision correct?

Mary is a 72-year-old woman who was admitted to hospital with right-arm weakness and difficulty speaking. She was diagnosed as having had a stroke and was admitted to the hospital's stroke unit. Routine blood tests showed evidence of some damage to the heart muscle and her electrocardiogram was also somewhat abnormal. Her doctors sent her to the cardiac catheterization laboratory for coronary angiography.

Were the doctors correct in ordering this invasive diagnostic procedure?

Each of these stories represents possible interactions between patients and their doctors that could occur in any office or hospital setting. By now, most readers probably suspect that the decisions which were taken were not the correct ones. These are but a few of many examples where beliefs held by either patients or physicians may seem logical but are not necessarily supported by scientific evidence. In the following pages, you will see how research studies involving actual patients can provide answers not only to the above questions, but also insights into other aspects of our health and the perils of daily living. However, I will first introduce the topic of medical research and how I came to be a participant in this evolving field.

In 1921, Dr. Fredrick Banting and Charles Best discovered insulin while working in the basement of an old building at the University of Toronto. At the time, Best was only a medical student spending his summer helping out on a research project, which probably explains why he didn't share in the Nobel Prize given to Banting and another colleague, J.J. MacLeod. Today, major discoveries in medicine usually involve teams of highly experienced scientists in research institutes using complex technology to achieve what are often modest advances in knowledge. Multiple advances are then combined to create a major discovery, with many scientists having participated along the way. Grants for supporting medical research are now mostly awarded to teams of specialists, sometimes working in different cities or even countries, whose members combine their expertise to achieve important advances in patient care. When I began my research career in medicine in 1972, Charles Best was still active and it was possible for an independent researcher working in modest surroundings to achieve significant breakthroughs. Although the conditions for performing research in medicine and its related fields may have become more complex, there is still an important role for the individual investigator who can see gaps in our knowledge that require further study. Even if subsequent studies are performed by a group of investigators, the ideas for studies often still come from one person.

In today's world, medical research is perhaps the most visible example of scientific discovery. Yet new ideas are equally important in many different fields involving innovation. A medical researcher discovering a new treatment is not much different than an automobile engineer developing a safety device which reduces traffic accidents. Education may be a common path to success, but other factors are just as important when it comes to conceiving original ideas. In fact, the top students in school are not necessarily the most successful innovators in later life. Other life experiences, such as learning to cope with adversity, being different from one's peers, and exposure to a variety of viewpoints can be very useful in recognizing opportunities for studies.

Looking back on the five decades of my career in medicine, I can identify several influences beyond education which led me to conduct a wide variety of research studies, many having direct relevance to our everyday lives. My success was mostly dependent on being able to question what others took for granted and to see gaps in our knowledge which had previously gone unnoticed. These skills were not learned in a classroom or from a book, but instead evolved, starting from my childhood experiences related to being different. Humans are not unlike other animal species in wanting to be part of the herd. Not being accepted by one's classmates can have a negative and often permanent impact on one's perceptions. Alternatively, learning how to overcome these obstacles may lead to positive outcomes in later life. I always knew that my childhood was different than most, but it took many years for me to realize that being different was not all bad. In fact, it may have been an asset when it later came to evaluating generally accepted beliefs, which were often based more on conjecture than on fact.

I shall begin the story of my career in medical research by providing some details of my family background and how growing up in Toronto as the first child of immigrants likely contributed to my success in later life. Thereafter, I shall describe my involvement in more than 60 studies covering a wide range of topics. Some studies are described in greater detail than others and a few probably contain scientific terms that some readers may find difficult to understand, despite my best efforts to use non-medical language. If, this happens, simply skip over to the next one. The remaining 59 should be more easily understood.

There are two sections which should be of special interest. The first is a rather detailed account of my libel suit against the Canadian Broadcasting Corporation related to my studies on the treatment of high blood pressure. The last part of the book describes how my research is changing how doctors around the world measure blood pressure in their offices. By the final page, readers should be able to see how opportunities for discovery exist in all areas of research. They are simply waiting for someone to find them.

But first, I will start with a brief account of my years before medicine in order to provide some insight into how this period influenced my future career.

ONE

The Early Years

I was born and raised in Toronto. My parents had arrived in Canada as teen-agers in the 1920s. they met about 15 years later and were married in 1945, two months before I was born. They must have both been quite 'modern' to be living together in sin in the 1940s, only deciding to marry so that I would become 'legitimate'. Already I was different than my future playmates, but I only learned about this part of my story many years later.

Both of my parents had been raised in orthodox Jewish homes in central Europe. By the 1930s, my mother had become a member of the Commu-nist Party of Canada. She had left the restaurant in Winnipeg where she was working as a waitress to see a demonstration in the street. Someone pinned a red button on her and when she returned to the restaurant, she was fired by her boss for being a communist. During the depression, there were plenty of communists in the north end of Winnipeg, so my mother had lots of com-pany. As for my father, I'm not sure of his political views in the 1930s but, in later life, I would say he was an 'arm-chair socialist'. He had developed an antipathy to joining organizations. Instead, he had an insatiable appetite for learning about the world, past and present.

Many Jewish immigrants to Canada had limited formal education, al-though they had often been raised in an environment which encouraged learning and individual effort. At the time, there was widespread anti-Semi-tism in much of Europe. In countries such as Poland and the Ukraine where my parents had lived, Jews were excluded from most of the business world and the professions. As a result, many were tradesmen, with the more for-tunate becoming writers, musicians and actors. The role of women mostly centered on looking after the home. My father left Poland after finishing high school, where he had also been exposed to many of the great European au-thors, scientists and performers, some of whom were Jewish. Once in Canada, he became an avid reader, which led to a life-long process of self-education. As in many Jewish immigrant families, education was of paramount importance.

One reason for mentioning my family background is to draw attention to the fact that immigrants and their children in Canada and the United States are often quite successful in later life. For instance, most Nobel Prize winners in the United States were either immigrants themselves or the children of immigrants. As the son of immigrants, I may also have benefitted from my background.

Even in being Jewish, I was still different from the other Jewish children in our neighbourhood. We weren't religious and didn't celebrate the Jewish holidays. My parents belonged to a secular, left-wing Jewish organization, which was still quite active in the 1950s. As part of its children's program, I was taken to Charlie Chaplin movies, saw the famous mime Marcel Marceau, met Paul Robeson and had several singing lessons from Pete Seeger. At the age of 10, I had a speaking role in a play before an audience of 500. At age 13, I gave a speech to a thousand people on behalf of the youth division of my parents' organization at its 25th anniversary celebration. My early years were far different from those of my playmates. Like Thurber's Walter Mitty, I had a secret life.

Many of my parents' friends who shared their political views also had children, which gave me a second group of playmates, separate from those at school or in the neighbourhood. In retrospect, I was not the only one whose future may have benefited from being different. Some became famous as singers, actors, artists, university professors and even mainstream politicians. After all, a Communist Party member of the Ontario Legislature, A.A. MacLeod, in later years became an advisor to John Robarts, the leader of the Conservative Party, who was the Premier of Ontario. Being different didn't seem to affect his future and may even have been an asset.

By now, you must be wondering what any of this have has to do with medical research. Nothing in itself, but probably a lot for me. Not being the same as my friends likely caused me to see my surroundings from a different perspective. Perhaps this may be the 'immigrant advantage' which my parents bestowed on me. Regardless of its origins, this quality became a useful asset later in my career.

My early years in grade school were not especially noteworthy. Somewhere between the third and fourth grade, I went from being average to standing first in the class. When this happened again in Grade 5, I ended up skipping a year, landing in Grade 7. I then returned to being an average student. Going from one of the older children in the class to the youngest also required some adjustment on my part.

In 1958, the high schools in Toronto undertook an experiment which involved having the top students entering Grade 9 complete the first four years of high school in three, followed by a full year of Grade 13 before graduation. My classroom in Grade 8 was split, with only 12 Grade 8 students and the others being in Grade 7. Somehow, the teacher taught both years in the same room. There was one other class composed only of Grade 8 students. Each of the five elementary schools which sent pupils to Grade 9 at Bloor Collegiate was able to select one or two students for the special 'accelerated' class. The remaining pupils were chosen on the basis of IQ tests, which were given to everyone in Grade 8. Somehow, seven of the twelve in our class, myself included, ended up in the special class of 33 students at Bloor Collegiate. No wonder I had felt 'average' in my Grade 8 class.

Thus, I began my four years of high school, graduating three months after turning 17, which made me two years younger than most of the others in my grade. My marks were satisfactory, but not exceptional. In retrospect, I think I was intelligent enough to do better, but was hampered by my relative youth. This view is supported by my grades in the final term of Grade 13, which were the best of my years in high school. I suppose my concentration improved when I knew that the marks would determine my future, such as being accepted into the university course of my choice—medicine. Without going into further detail, I can now see how being different and also younger than my peers had a major negative impact on my four years in high school. I had no regrets in leaving Bloor Collegiate behind.

TWO

Medical School and Internship

Medicine had not been my first choice for a future career. I liked chemistry and thought about becoming a chemical engineer, even though I had never met one and knew little about what it involved. My plans soon changed after my father pointed out that there were almost no Jewish engineers, which was certainly true in 1962. My next thought was of becoming a veterinarian, but I progressed to medicine when I discovered that the course for looking after people was only one year longer. After all, I was young enough to spend the additional year in university.

I graduated from medical school at the University of Toronto in 1968. My standing in the class was mostly 'average'. I can honestly say that nothing I ever did in medical school was in any way noteworthy. By the time of graduation, I did have one clear goal—to do my internship somewhere other than in Toronto, the city in which I was born and until then, where I had spent my entire life.

The year before my graduation had been a continuous celebration of Canada's centennial, with the Expo 67 World's Fair in Montreal as its focal point. When it came to the selection of a hospital for internship, Canada had a national program which matched applicants to positions, based mostly on academic performance at the end of the third year of medical school. Once again, my best marks in university were achieved when I most needed them. They were good enough to get me an internship at my first choice, the Montreal General Hospital. It was no longer the centennial year, but Montreal after Expo 67 was still very attractive for someone of my age.

My year of internship was full of contradictions. The first four months on the internal medicine service were sheer hell. I was on call every second night, which meant sleeping only several hours. One time when my partner went on holidays, I was on call eight out of nine nights, probably the worst nine days of my life. I have no idea how I was able to function in my sleep-deprived state. Somehow, I survived these first four months of being a doctor.

The other rotations were much more tolerable. In fact, I was off-call entirely during my two-month rotation in pediatrics at the Montreal Children's Hospital. Besides one francophone, I was the only one of 15 anglophone interns who would see French-speaking children in the outpatient clinic. One of my reasons for being in Montreal was to improve my high-school French. The McGill University graduates seemed to have little interest in speaking French. It was not too difficult to understand why separation from English Canada was becoming so popular in Quebec.

I was supposed to spend my second month of the pediatric rotation working on the wards in the hospital. However, because of my improving linguistic skills, I was asked to remain in the outpatient clinic. By then, having a Quebecoise nurse as a girlfriend had further advanced my linguistic education. Besides being exposed to French-Canadian culture, the other highlight of my stay was learning how to ski, which is what everyone in Montreal seemed to do on weekends from November until April.

At year's end, interns at the Montreal General Hospital were required to undergo an 'exit interview', in my case conducted by two senior physicians in the Department of Medicine, who had been at the hospital since before World War ll. From my perspective, it seemed that they had been there since the hospital opened in 1821.

The interview began with a question: Why had I been rated one of the worst interns in years during my four months on internal medicine at the Montreal General Hospital and one of the best interns during my two months at the Montreal Children's Hospital and at the Catherine Booth Hospital (where I had done my rotation in obstetrics)? I proceeded to relate my experiences on call, working without sleep, recording electrocardiograms with machines made of wood, starting all the intravenous lines for patients and taking their blood samples every morning. I could have also mentioned that all of the hospital's requisitions for tests had a line at the bottom which said 'signature of doctor or intern'. Somehow the institution did not recognize that all of the interns were already doctors of medicine. This one line said everything. Compared to the hospitals in Toronto, the working conditions on the internal medicine wards were medieval. But June 15 finally arrived and I had survived the year.

THREE

Residency in Internal Medicine

After my final year of medical school, I had developed a plan for what was to follow. My classmates were either proceeding into residency programs for different specialties or into family practice in the community. Being different, I had other ideas. After internship, I would work in Toronto for six months as a family doctor and then travel around the world for the next six months. Upon returning, I would do one year of residency in internal medicine, before setting up practice as a family doctor, somewhere in the Toronto area. With this combination, my medical training would provide me with the skills needed for my future professional life, whereas my experiences during the six months of travel would satisfy my curiosity to see more of the world.

As fate would have it, I never got the opportunity to see the outcome of my plan. Yes, I did travel for six months and then successfully applied for a residency position. What I didn't anticipate was a series of opportunities which would lead me to a career in medical research.

The first one occurred in October 1970, three months after the start of my residency in internal medicine at the Toronto Western Hospital. The head of the Department of Medicine, Dr. Irwin Hilliard, was a traditional academic who was both a superb physician and an excellent teacher of post-graduate trainees. He had come to know me when I had been his resident on the private medicine service in July, during my first month at the hospital. One day in October, he invited me into his office for a friendly chat, as was sometimes his custom. But on this occasion, he asked about my plans for the following year. I told him that I intended to go into family practice in Toronto, using the additional experience from my year of internal medicine to help me look after more complex cases. To my surprise, he said that I had been doing an excellent job and that he wanted me to remain for a second year of training. I was dumbfounded. At this point, I was only just starting to feel comfortable after three months as a resident. Six months of being away from patients had taken its toll. After several minutes of being told how well I was doing, I began to feel more at ease and said I would consider his offer.

Not since my teacher in Grade 5 had promoted me to Grade 7 had anyone ever been so positive about my potential. Dr. Hilliard must have noticed something beyond my knowledge of medicine, which was certainly not as deep as many of the other residents. I don't recall exactly what I thought about the offer, nor the question of what I would do after a second year of training. What I do know is that I accepted the offer and remained at the hospital for another year.

As the months went by, my interests began to drift away from family practice. However, I could not see myself spending several more years to become a specialist in internal medicine. Once again, I had become restless and wanted a change in venue from the city of my birth. Coincidentally, a new centre for the treatment of drug addiction that had just opened in Toronto had attracted my attention. I soon thought about doing a research fellowship in neuropharmacology, with a view to becoming a clinical pharmacologist, in my case specializing in the treatment of addiction to drugs. I suppose my interests came from my exposure to clinical pharmacology at the Montreal General Hospital, where a young clinical pharmacologist, Dr. John Ruedy, had impressed me because of his superb clinical skills and research interests. Unfortunately, my experience at the Montreal General precluded any thought I might have had about returning there.

I proceeded to apply to several clinical pharmacology programs in the United States and one at the Hammersmith Hospital in London, England. By chance, I learned that Colin Dollery, the professor of clinical pharmacology at the Hammersmith Hospital, was coming to McMaster University's Medical School in nearby Hamilton in March for a short sabbatical. He invited me to visit him there to discuss my interest in working in his department. I spoke about wanting to do research in neuropharmacology. He told me that several members of his department were already doing work involving the brain, but the main focus of this research was examining how various drugs might lower blood pressure by acting on the central nervous system. The study of high blood pressure (hypertension) was much closer to cardiology and had nothing to do with addiction. By chance, I also had developed an interest in cardiology, after my father had undergone heart surgery in 1967.

As I had already exhausted my options when it came to doing clinical pharmacology elsewhere, it was time to make a decision. It didn't take long for me to conclude that the opportunity to spend a year in London doing research in hypertension was more attractive than returning to my original plan of going into family practice. After a brief conversation, Professor Dollery offered me a research position with the understanding that it did not include any salary. I had already considered this possibility and had concluded that a year without funding would be possible, but only if I worked in a family practice during the summer and saved my money. I accepted his offer, with the intention of starting my research training at the beginning of September.

According to plan, I found a *locum tenens* position with three family doctors in Port Credit, near Toronto. They all did shifts in the emergency department of the nearby hospital and were quite happy to let me replace them, so that they could spend more time at the cottage, enjoying the pleasant summer weather. I was somewhat surprised by how much I enjoyed my work in family practice. Also, my income from the extra shifts in the emergency department would make surviving in London much easier. By the end of the summer, I had decided that I would accept their invitation for me to join their practice if my plans for London didn't work out.

Next, I decided to visit Dr. Douglas Wigle, head of the University of Toronto's cardiology program, to discuss the possibility of getting a position as a resident in cardiology upon my return from London the following summer. Once again, I was given an unexpected opportunity. Wigle and Dollery had trained together at the Hammersmith in the late 1950s. Wigle had thought quite highly of his co-worker and was impressed that I had obtained a research position in his department. He also had contacts at the Ontario Heart Foundation and, with his support, I found myself with a two-year research fellowship for training in hypertension. I now had ample funds to survive in London, which turned out to be a lot more expensive than I had anticipated.

At this point, I had come to accept that my path to medical practice would be much longer than I had originally planned. My future was now shifting more to an academic appointment at a teaching hospital. Today, the required training would include an undergraduate university degree followed by four years of medical school, three years of residency in general internal medicine, two to three years of clinical training in a sub-specialty, and then several years of research, often leading to a Ph.D. A graduate from high school could now be looking at 15 years or more of training. Once again, I was able to 'skip' a few years. For me, it was only 11 years, including university and my rotating internship, not because I was some kind of prodigy, but because of the accident of my date of birth, it being in 1945 and not 30 or more years later. Needless to say, we are now in a different era when it comes to training for a career in medical research. Even in 1970, my path to a research position at a university teaching hospital was unusually short.

FOUR

Training in Research with Rabbits and Rats

I arrived at the Hammersmith Hospital at the beginning of September 1972 and was assigned to work with Dr. John Reid, Senior Registrar (Senior Resident), and Dr. Peter Lewis, Registrar (Resident), in the Department of Clinical Pharmacology. The latter had recently replaced Dr. John Chalmers, a visiting professor from Australia who had introduced a specialized technique for injecting tiny amounts of liquids into the brains of rabbits and rats. There was not a single patient in sight, only New Zealand White rabbits and Wistar rats. Working solely with animals was certainly not something I had anticipated, but I had no choice. There were about 1,500 doctors at the Hammersmith and only 500 patients! When senior registrars and registrars were not involved in their research, they were spending several months each year looking after patients on the wards. I was not there for clinical training and the number of patients available for research was quite limited. So, rabbits and rats it would be for the next 12 months.

By December 1972, I had completed my apprenticeship in animal research. I had learned to use tiny screws to attach plastic plates to the skulls of rabbits. The small plates had holes which lined up with liquid-filled chambers inside the small brains of the animals, called ventricles. Using a fine needle, we were able to inject tiny amounts of various drugs and chemicals into the (cerebral) ventricles to see if they might cause changes in the animal's blood pressure and pulse rate which were measured using a small-diameter catheter placed into an artery in the ear.

At the time of my arrival, the main drug of interest in the laboratory was propranolol, a relatively new medication being used to treat high blood pressure. There were two reasons for injecting small amounts of propranolol into the fluid in the cerebral ventricles of the rabbits. First, it was known from studies using radioactive propranolol that the drug was highly concentrated in the brains of animals compared to the concentration in the blood. Second, blood pressure is partly controlled by impulses sent out from the brain via sympathetic nerves to the heart and circulation. Since propranolol decreased both heart rate and blood pressure, it might have several actions, including a reduction in impulses sent from the brain to these sympathetic nerves. We already had a technique for injecting substances into the (cerebrospinal) fluid in the brain, so we proceeded to investigate this possibility in the rabbit model.

Although I was the most junior member of our group, both my colleagues were very helpful in teaching me the required techniques so that I could soon conduct experiments of my own. Sure enough, increasing doses of propranolol did seem to reduce the blood pressure of rabbits, including those with both normal and high readings.

The British Pharmacological Society held scientific meetings several times a year. By early 1973, I had enough new data to include in an abstract for submission to the March 28 meeting in Leeds. The abstract (1) was accepted, which meant that I next had to prepare 10 to 12 slides for a 10-minute presentation. (Numbers in parentheses indicate an item in the list of references at the end of the book.) In our department, it was customary for presenters to rehearse before all the members of the department. These sessions had a reputation for being far worse than the actual presentation. My maiden effort was no exception. My slides were criticized, my verbal description of the content was deficient and I was told not to read so much from my notes. With the help of my co-workers, John and Peter, l was able to revise the slides. I learned to put the text of my presentation on the slides in point form, so that I could read each point as a sentence. In doing so, my eyes would be looking toward the audience instead of down at a piece of paper.

I recall being the second or third presenter on the first morning of the meeting. As soon as I started to speak, the microphone went dead. There were several hundred people in the audience, so I could not proceed without it. After a short delay, I was given a replacement microphone to hold in my hand, leaving my other hand for the electric pointer. Suddenly, I was one hand short! I needed both hands to advance the slides and adjust the file cards on the podium. (They contained brief notes to be used, if needed.) Somehow, I made it through the talk. In fact, after the session, I received several compliments from my colleagues. The presentation must have surprised them, since the rehearsal had been so dreadful. Sometimes it's helpful to begin with low expectations.

Next, it was back to the Hammersmith to see how the rabbits were doing. By now, I was somewhat surprised that it was possible to be excited about doing research with animals. Together with John and Peter, I continued with my experiments, injecting tiny amounts of propranolol into the cerebrospinal fluid inside the ventricle of the brain. Our studies confirmed that the drug did have an effect on the sympathetic nervous system that could be responsible for its blood pressure lowering action.

The next task was to prepare a manuscript outlining our findings for submission to the *Journal of Pharmacology and Experimental Therapeutics*. Since I had been designated as the lead investigator on this project, the task of writing the manuscript was given over to me. I clearly recall writing seven drafts of the paper with each one being reviewed by Peter and John. Seven times, I received feedback on what I had written, including recommendations for changes. Finally, John took my last draft, changed the order of several paragraphs, added in a few sentences here and there and returned the "final" version of the manuscript to me.

It looked much better, except for one problem. John had now put his own name first, indicating that he was the senior author. I tried hard not to show my disappointment, since I had been looking forward to seeing my first publication. However, John had supervised all of my work and the experiments had been his idea. He anticipated that this change in authorship would bother me and put me somewhat at ease by reminding me that there would soon be other opportunities to be the senior author on research articles. I could not disagree and also was grateful for all the time he had devoted to educating me on how to write a scientific paper. By now, I had learned more about the English system for training researchers. There were no formal courses. Instead, there was excellent mentorship with one-to-one teaching. Within a few weeks, our manuscript was accepted for publication (2).

My initial work with the rat population involved holding the creatures for John, so that he could monitor their response to substances which he administered to them. This important role got me a credit as a co-author on his next article.

My only experiment with Wistar rats involved injecting a substance called 5,6-dihydroxy-tryptamine (5,6-DHT) into their cerebrospinal fluid in the brain. 5,6-DHT was known to destroy cells in the brain which contained a substance called serotonin. Our interest in propranolol's effects on the brain led us to examine the possible role serotonin might play in the regulation of blood pressure. (Serotonin is also the substance which the antidepressant Prozac inhibits.) The idea was to see if destroying these serotonin-containing cells would prevent the development of hypertension, which occurs when rats are treated with DOCA-saline (a combination of the steroid, deoxycorti-costerone acetate, and a high sodium diet). The control group was only given a small amount of salt solution. The results of the experiment were negative. The destruction of the serotonergic cells did not prevent the development of hypertension. (Since we were unable to determine if the rats had become less depressed, we missed out on discovering a possible treatment for depression.)

The brief mention of this experiment involving rats provides an opportunity for me to tell what happened next. I prepared an abstract describing this somewhat disappointing experiment and submitted it for possible presentation at the annual meeting of the European Society for Clinical Investigation, which, at the time, was a major international meeting. I was the senior author, with John Reid and Peter Lewis as co-authors, since they had helped with the experiments. It was also customary to have the name of Professor Colin Dollery on all presentations and publications from the department. However, he had not been very impressed by the results of this experiment and asked that his name not be included as a co-author. As luck would have it, the abstract was not only accepted for presentation, but was also selected for the opening plenary session. Somebody must have thought the findings were of interest. The meeting was at the end of April in Rotterdam, Holland. There were at least 500 attendees in the audience. Even a hundred would have made me quite nervous. Fortunately, it was 13 months after my first presentation in Leeds and I was now a more confident and capable speaker.

The chair of the session was Professor Alberto Zanchetti from Milan, who at the age of 46 was already recognized as a leader in hypertension research. After I finished speaking, he proceeded to ask me a question about several aspects of the transmission of impulses in the brain from the work of Dr. Alfred Sjoerdsma. At this point, I should clarify that if I were now an "expert," it was only in my very narrow area of research. I had heard of Dr. Sjoerdsma, but was not very familiar with his work.

I stood at the podium trying my best to look intelligent without knowing how to respond. Dr. Zanchetti soon came to my rescue by proceeding to answer his own question, saying "I think you would agree that…" His delivery was so smooth that many in the audience probably thought that it was

I who had answered the question. Dr. Zanchetti was a true gentleman and I never forgot that moment when he had saved me from certain embarrassment. Over the next 45 years, I had many opportunities to meet with him to discuss various research activities. He was still the editor of the *Journal of Hypertension* in 2018 when, at age 91, he stumbled on the stairs in his house and sustained a fatal head injury.

I have included this experiment to show how a career in research can have many different facets. Although the findings were negative, others must have found serotonin's not having a role in the development of hypertension of interest. An article based on these experiments was sent to *Cardiovascular Research* for possible publication. Within a week, the manuscript had been favourably reviewed by two experts and I was told that it had been accepted. This success was noteworthy in that Professor Dollery was not listed as a co-author (his own wish). It was good to know that even professors were not always right when it came to predicting the interest in our experiments.

Meanwhile, I was still thinking about humans and how our findings in rabbits and rats could be relevant to patients with hypertension. You may recall that my first experiment involved injecting propranolol into the brains of rabbits. I would soon have an opportunity to examine the effects of this drug in greater detail, not only in rabbits, but also humans.

FIVE

Propranolol and Paraquat Poisoning

I may not have been on the Dean's List in medical school, but I must have developed other skills which, until then, were unknown to me. I was about to benefit from recognizing an opportunity which others did not see. This one was to be the first of many.

The story of my career in research now moves from rabbits and rats to a dog. As we were completing the experiments injecting propranolol into the brains of rabbits, an opportunity appeared which was to make the findings in animals more relevant to humans. The drug we had been studying, propranolol, is composed of 2 parts, called 'd' and 'l' isomers. The molecular structure of each isomer is the mirror image of the other, but only the l-isomer of propranolol is responsible for its pharmacologic effect, the inhibition of sympathetic nervous system activity, which is how the drug lowers blood pressure. However, both isomers had other properties, including a local anesthetic effect which was thought to be of little consequence in humans.

At this time, there had been several reports of people being accidentally poisoned by a weed killer called Paraquat. After ingestion, Paraquat attacked the tissue of the lungs, with the unlucky patient dying slowly over a period of several weeks. Investigators in Scotland had performed some preliminary experiments which suggested that local anesthetic agents, such as d-propranolol, might interfere with the binding of Paraquat to the lung tissue. d-Propranolol was especially attractive, since it was otherwise relatively harmless, even at higher concentrations, and could be administered intravenously. Given that the Hammersmith Hospital was a national centre for medical research, arrangements were made to have future patients with Paraquat poisoning transferred to our institution for treatment with d-propranolol.

Several of the senior staff in our department were acting as consultants to the doctors in the Intensive Care Unit because of their knowledge of drugs and, more specifically, of propranolol. After the first patient treated with d-propranolol died, I saw an opportunity to reproduce our studies in rabbits, without having to infuse propranolol into the brain of humans. Before proceeding any further, I should explain that the practice of obtaining written informed consent from patients or their relatives before performing any human experimentation was not nearly as rigorous in 1973 as it is today. In view of what follows, I don't recall personally meeting with any of the patients' relatives, although other members of our department probably did so. Since what I was about to do was relatively harmless, I suspect that my actions were considered to be benign.

I was able to complement the experiments we had done in the rabbits by obtaining data on the ratio of the amount of d-propranolol in the human brain to its concentration in blood. I was notified of the transfer of the next five patients admitted with Paraquat poisoning who, by the time I saw them, had been started on intravenous d-propranolol. I visited them daily to monitor their progress and to take periodic samples of blood to follow the concentration of d-propranolol. There was a therapeutic aspect to my actions in that propranolol is metabolized in the liver and its concentration in the blood can vary tenfold among different individuals. Knowing the concentration in the blood allowed the doctors to adjust the dose of the drug to produce what was considered to be the optimum benefit. Having these results also turned out to be quite useful for my research.

Unfortunately, d-propranolol was ineffective in stopping the damage to lung tissue caused by the Paraquat and all five patients died. The attempt to change an otherwise fatal outcome had unfortunately been unsuccessful. I had arranged to be present at each of the autopsies and was given a small piece of brain tissue for analysis of its d-propranolol content. Since I already had the matching blood samples, it was now possible to calculate the brain to blood ratio of d-propranolol as we had done in rabbits using dl-propranolol. The ratios were comparable to what we had seen in the rabbit experiments since the d- and l-isomers were otherwise identical. These findings showed that propranolol achieved high concentrations in the brain of both rabbits and humans, which supported the concept that the drug might decrease blood pressure by acting on the central nervous system. An article based upon these experiments was published in the *Journal of Pharmacology and Experimental Therapeutics* (4), this time with me as the senior author. John Reid had kept his word.

Earlier, I mentioned a dog had played a role in these investigations. No, the dog did not help us to discover a new aspect of propranolol's action, nor did it help us to find a treatment for hypertension.

An astute intern, who took the history from one of the five patients, noted that the family dog had died shortly before his owner had become ill. In this case, the patient did not know how he had come to ingest the Paraquat. He frequently worked in his garden and did use Paraquat as a weed-killer. Perhaps he had ingested it by accident, since he sometimes kept the Paraquat in a household bottle in the garden shed.

The intern who first saw the patient wondered if the poisoning and death of the family dog might be related. He reported his suspicions to his supervisor who then notified the police. When they exhumed the body of the dog from its burial site in the backyard of the family home, they found that the dog's tissues contained a very high concentration of Paraquat. After further enquiries, the source of the patient's poisoning became clear. His wife had been having an extra-marital affair and conspired with her lover to put small amounts of Paraquat into her husband's food, such that the amount in his body had increased to the point where it ultimately became fatal. The poor dog was being fed the scraps from the family meals and had also died of Paraquat poisoning. Fortunately, the guilty couple did not have to journey very far. The famous Wormwood Scrubs Prison was located beside the hospital, so that the felons might have sometimes been able to see the roof of the hospital building where the poor husband had died.

Looking back at these events, I recognize the role that opportunity had played in these experiments. First, I overcame the initial disappointment of having to work with animals and then saw an opportunity to perform my first human experiment, though it was somewhat macabre, even by the standards of 1973. One might ask about the importance of knowing that a drug achieves high concentrations in the brain. In this instance, this finding provided an explanation for some of propranolol's side effects, especially nightmares and other disturbances of brain function. Subsequent beta-blocking drugs (see atenolol in next section) did not exhibit these adverse effects because they did not cross from the blood into brain tissue. Thus, a somewhat esoteric finding can be of importance, especially if you are a patient who is experiencing a side effect. Yes, what you are feeling may truly be "only in your head."

SIX

My First Clinical Trial

I continued with my animal studies until the summer of 1973, when I returned to Toronto for a brief, two-week holiday. Once back at the Hammersmith, I was finally asked to work in the Hypertension Clinic. Since John Reid had gone to the National Institutes of Health in Bethesda to work with the Nobel laureate Julius Axelrod and Peter Lewis had begun to prepare his Ph.D. thesis, I had now become the "senior" member of our hypertension research team. Progress in academic medicine in England was certainly not glacial. By now, I seem to have been recognized as an expert in beta-blockers, the class of drugs to which propranolol belonged. My "graduation" to expert may have occurred when a professor in medicine at the University of Oxford called me on the telephone to ask my opinion about a patient with hypertension who was having a problem with his medications, one of which was propranolol.

My participation in the Hypertension Clinic also gave me the opportunity to become involved in research with real patients and not just rabbits and rats. The Department of Clinical Pharmacology had a national reputation for research into new medications for treating hypertension. At this time, Imperial Chemical Industries (ICI) was involved in many areas, including the manufacture of household paints, various chemicals and pharmaceutical products. Several years before, they had developed propranolol, first for the treatment of angina and later for hypertension. Propranolol was the first beta-blocker drug approved for use in humans and was soon followed by a sister drug called practolol, also a beta-blocker. In September 1973, ICI approached Professor Dollery with a proposal to study a third beta-blocker, at this point called ICI-66082, as a possible treatment for hypertension.

I would like to say that I was the first person asked to do the study. Alas, I was probably number three in the queue. Two of the more senior researchers who had been training in the department for several years turned down the opportunity to study ICI-66082. Since there were already two beta-blockers on the market, propranolol and practolol, they didn't see any likelihood of there being yet another. What none of us knew at the time was that practolol would be withdrawn from the market several years later because of a serious adverse effect. ICI-66082, later called atenolol, would go on to become the most widely prescribed beta-blocker in the world. At the time, all I saw was an opportunity to be the lead investigator in a clinical trial involving real patients. Thus, I was able to do the first randomized, placebo-controlled trial of atenolol in hypertension.

I met with Professor Dollery who provided the outline for a possible study. After further discussions, we decided on the following approach. Patients with hypertension of "moderate" severity when not on medication were to be eligible for enrollment into the study. In 1973, moderate hypertension was defined as a diastolic blood pressure of 105 mmHg or greater. (Blood pressure is recorded as the highest and lowest pressures inside the artery with each heartbeat—the higher reading being the systolic and the lower one the diastolic blood pressure, both shown in terms of millimeters of mercury [mmHg]). The average reading in the participants at entry was 187/114 mmHg. Today, if a patient walked into an emergency department with such a reading, treatment would be considered urgent.

Each subject was to receive increasing doses of atenolol from 75 mg to 900 mg per day, if tolerated, in three divided doses of 25 to 300 mg, with increments in dosage being made every two weeks. Once the optimum dose was reached (blood pressure response versus side effects), patients were randomly allocated to eight weeks of treatment with both this dose and a matching placebo, the order of the two "treatments" being decided by chance. Thus, some patients received only 25 mg of atenolol three times a day, whereas a few others attained the maximum dose of 300 mg thrice daily. At the end of this "run-in" period, eight patients were taking a total of 300 mg daily and six were receiving 600 mg daily. Note that all subjects were off therapy for eight weeks during the placebo phase of the trial, despite some having a very high blood pressure at entry. Patients with such readings would never receive a placebo for eight weeks in a clinical trial today, but this was 1973, when it was not unusual to see patients with a blood pressure of 220/120 mmHg. It was certainly a different era back then.

Atenolol did lower blood pressure, but unexpectedly, it achieved its maximum effect in most patients at the starting dose of 25 mg three times a day.

Even though the majority of patients tolerated the higher doses, there was little additional decrease in blood pressure, but side effects were more common. The anti-hypertensive effects of atenolol in comparison with the placebo were confirmed in the second phase of the study.

There was one interesting side effect reported. During the 16-week treatment/placebo phase, one patient noted a recurrence of his migraine headaches two weeks after being switched from one study drug to the other. He said that he had not experienced a single migraine headache during the previous eight weeks. He asked if he was now on a placebo, since his headaches had returned. At the end of the study, we broke the code and discovered that his headaches had disappeared while on atenolol. This finding was reported in the publication on the study's results (5), but it would be quite a few years before the beneficial effects of beta-blockers as a prophylactic therapy for migraine would be recognized. Since atenolol did not cross into brain tissue, the importance of this observation was not obvious.

Just before my return to Toronto in June 1974, I was invited to the headquarters of ICI at Macclesfield, in northern England, to present the findings of my study. The audience consisted of senior researchers in pharmaceutical products at ICI, statisticians and marketing executives. The main point of my talk was that the atenolol was effective at the lowest dose of 25 mg three times a day, with only a few patients benefitting from the next higher dose. When I finished my presentation, there was a brief period of silence until several of the senior researchers began to question the validity of my findings.

I was then told that the company was planning to market the drug at a dose of 100 mg three times a day. As my study had only included 16 patients, I could not present a very forceful argument in support of my data. All I could say was that these were the observations I had made. It is interesting that it was possible to identify a major error in the proposed dosage for the drug in a study involving so few patients. Atenolol proceeded to be initially marketed at a dose of 100-200 mg once daily for the treatment of hypertension. By then, three times daily dosing had been found to be unnecessary.

Within a few years, atenolol became the most widely prescribed beta-blocker, surpassing propranolol, with the usual dose being 25–50 mg, once daily, with only a few patients receiving 100 mg once daily. Even today, it is still a popular beta-blocker in many countries.

So, my first clinical trial (5) involving only 16 patients had been a success, even though its findings were not recognized for several years. I should mention that the concept of doing clinical studies to determine the optimum dose of drugs, such as those used to treat hypertension, was relatively new. For example, nobody had ever done a similar study with propranolol and its recommended dose varied from 160 mg to 960 mg daily! To be fair to the people at ICI, at least they had been interested in having a dose-response study done for atenolol.

SEVEN

Subsequent Dose-Response Studies

(My apologies for leaping into the future at this point. I thought it would be more meaningful to complete this topic now, rather than come back to it later on.)

A few years later, in 1978, I went on to perform a similar study with another beta-blocker, metoprolol (6). Once again, the most effective dose was lower than what its manufacturer thought it should be. Metoprolol had already been on the market in several European countries at a recommended dose of 100 mg or 200 mg twice daily. This dose was also proposed for Canadian patients, despite there being no supporting data. After my experience with atenolol, it didn't take me long to see another opportunity for a study.

This time I enrolled 34 hypertensive patients who received an initial dose of metoprolol 50 mg twice daily, to be increased to a maximum of 300 mg twice daily. The maximum blood pressure lowering effect was seen at doses of either 50 or 100 mg twice daily (see figure 1), with little additional fall in blood pressure at the higher doses. These lower doses soon became the standard for clinical practice, effectively reducing the cost of the drug to patients by one-half, since the company had expected that doses of 100 mg or 200 mg twice daily would be prescribed.

Propranolol had not been the only anti-hypertensive drug to have its dose based upon conjecture and not data. The diuretic ("water pill") hydrochlorothiazide had been the most widely used treatment for hypertension since its introduction in the 1960s. Yet, its dose was not based on any research studies. In the mid-1980s, I recognized this oversight, which led me to perform another dose-response study, in this case with doses of 25 mg, 50 mg and 100 mg once daily. The results were as before, with the most effective dose being the lowest, 25 mg daily, in most patients, with some individuals receiving a little additional benefit at 50 mg daily (7). These results subsequently contrib-

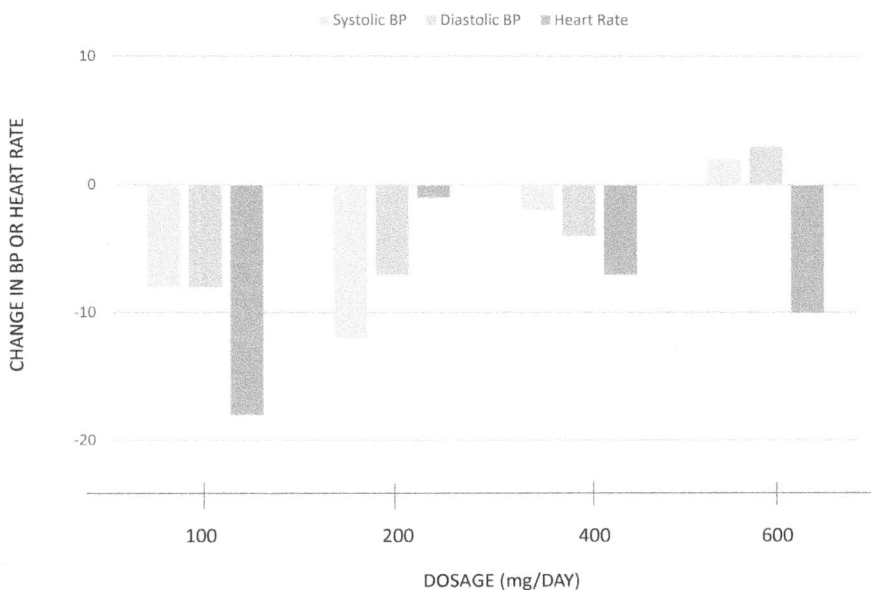

Figure 1. Changes in supine mean systolic and diastolic blood pressures (mm Hg) and heart rate (bpm) after long-term metopronol therapy at doses of 100 to 600 mg/day. Each set of values represents change in blood pressure or heart rate after previous dosage.

uted to a reduction in the dose of hydrochlorothiazide in clinical practice. Soon, very few patients were receiving the 100 mg dose, which was more likely to produce biochemical abnormalities in the blood such as a low potassium level.

I know for certain that these results did have a major impact on an important study which was being undertaken around this time. The Systolic Hypertension in the Elderly (SHEP) Trial was a study involving thousands of subjects over age 60 to determine if treating a systolic blood pressure of 160 mmHg or greater was beneficial. My role in this study developed by chance. Dr. McFate Smith, the principal investigator of the SHEP trial (8), and I were speaking on the same program at a meeting in Rio de Janeiro where I presented my hydrochlorothiazide dose-response data. After my talk, he approached me to discuss the pilot study he was then undertaking in order to demonstrate the feasibility of doing the much larger SHEP trial.

The treatment in the SHEP trial was another diuretic called chlorthalidone, which was similar to hydrochlorothiazide. Chlorthalidone had also been in use since the 1960s. Dr. Smith said the investigators were planning on using doses of 50 mg or 100 mg daily in the study patients, but he now wondered if lower doses might be better. He must have been impressed by my data, since he ended up reducing by one-half the dose of chlorthalidone in the SHEP trial. The trial was a great success (9) and today the dose of chlorthalidone in hypertension is usually even lower, 12.5 mg to 25 mg daily. Considering all the interest we have today in new drugs, it is remarkable that these two treatments for hypertension are still widely used after 60 years.

These dose-response studies were not difficult to perform, so it is surprising that it took so long for regulatory agencies, such as the Food and Drug Administration, to require that most new drugs, especially antihypertensive agents, undergo a proper dose-response evaluation early in their development. All of these dose-response studies had important implications for patient care. By decreasing the amount of medication by one-half or more, patients could reduce their likelihood of experiencing side-effects, avoid potentially harmful biochemical abnormalities and lower the costs of their treatment.

EIGHT

Returning to Canada from the Hammersmith

At the end of June 1974, I returned to Toronto to start my one year of residency in cardiology at Sunnybrook Hospital. Little did I know that 47 years later I would still be working there. During my time at Sunnybrook, its name changed several times, finally becoming Sunnybrook Health Sciences Centre. The hospital was initially built in the 1940s for veterans of World Wars l and II, but was transformed into a teaching hospital affiliated with the University of Toronto in 1966. Starting in the 1970s, a series of additions to the main building was constructed, and, by the 21st century, Sunnybrook Health Sciences Centre had more than doubled in size. A separate wing for the long-term care of veterans was also constructed, although in recent years, the number of World War ll veterans living there has gradually diminished.

During my year of training in cardiology I took my specialty examinations in Internal Medicine, even though a separate examination for cardiology had recently become available. Although I had been given credit for a year of cardiology training based upon my two years of research in hypertension at the Hammersmith, I was realistic in recognizing that I would not have passed the cardiology examination in November 1974, after less than six months of formal training in the specialty.

My main concern was passing the written portion of the internal medicine examination, which was usually taken after the completion of three to four years of residency training. Although I had studied during the evenings while in London, I was anxious about my chances of passing, especially since I had not been exposed to several sub-specialties in internal medicine. Also, at the Hammersmith, I had only been on-call four nights in two years, had not done any in-patient care and had only worked in the Hypertension Clinic once a week during my second year. Thus, when I arrived at Sunnybrook in July 1974, I had not performed a complete examination on a patient for almost two years.

I don't know what my mark was on the written examination, but it was good enough to pass, which allowed me to proceed to the next phase, the oral examination. If my experience at the Hammersmith had taught me one thing, it was how to think on my feet while under stress. During the two years, I had presented my research at least six times at both national and international scientific meetings. The rehearsals before each presentation were also quite helpful. So, when it came to the oral fellowship examination, I was reasonably confident of passing. My only concern was that the patients assigned for me to see might have conditions in the sub-specialties I had not been trained in. Fortunately, my three cases had either cardiac or respiratory problems and I had no difficulty in scoring a high mark, or so I was told by the chief examiner.

Now I could begin to look for a staff position at a university teaching hospital. For practical reasons, I wanted to remain in Toronto, if possible, since I was now married with a daughter soon to arrive. Also, by then, my appetite for travel and living abroad had been satisfied. From a clinical perspective, my training in cardiology was obviously deficient, in that I had only completed two years of internal medicine and was doing only one year of residency in cardiology. On the other hand, I had been the senior author on several scientific papers, which was impressive when compared to other applicants for staff positions in clinical research. Also, I was interested in hypertension, a field which attracted few specialists, despite being a very common condition. Moreover, the practice of cardiology was not nearly as complex as it is today.

When I first arrived at Sunnybrook as a resident, they were doing one heart catheterization a day compared to more than 20 today. Instead of a treadmill, three wooden steps were being used for exercise tests and there were no ultrasound tests or nuclear medicine studies of the heart. The hospital did have the most modern coronary care unit in the city, since it had only become a general hospital eight years earlier. However, cardiology was still a rather simple specialty back then. Patients with a heart attack were routinely put to bed and given morphine for any chest pain. The stay in intensive care usually lasted four to five days, followed by at least a week on the cardiology ward.

By March 1975, I had received an offer of an appointment from Sunnybrook, mainly because I was able to get a research scholarship from the Ontario Heart Foundation, which provided most of my salary for the next nine years. I also had a second offer at a smaller hospital doing mostly patient care with some research, if time permitted. Needless to say, I would not be writing this book today, had I not been successful in obtaining the Heart Foundation scholarship.

Although most of my year as a resident was devoted to training in clinical cardiology, I did get involved in some research. One of the younger staff cardiologists had trained in Montreal where he learned of a possible treatment for spasm of coronary arteries, which sometimes occurred during cardiac catheterization procedures. Some patients with coronary artery spasm had chest pain with otherwise normal coronary arteries, whereas others had fixed blockages due to deposits of cholesterol at the site of the spasm. These attacks often caused considerable distress, since they also tended to occur during daily activities and often mimicked a heart attack.

The second cardiac catheterization in which I participated involved a 50-year-old woman with recurrent chest pain suggestive of angina. The cardiologist immediately identified that her otherwise normal right and left coronary arteries were exhibiting spasm, which persisted even after the catheter had been withdrawn. He decided to test the possibility of preventing the spasm by injecting an old drug, phentolamine, into the coronary artery. This drug would theoretically prevent spasm of the muscular tissue in the arterial wall by blocking the stimulation of receptors which caused the vessel wall to constrict. As it turned out, the phentolamine had a dramatic effect in abolishing the catheter-induced spasm.

After observing the apparent success of this new treatment, I offered to prepare a brief article for possible publication in the *Canadian Medical Association Journal*. I quickly wrote and submitted a manuscript, which also included a picture of the artery, both in spasm and then without spasm after administration of the phentolamine. The submission was accepted and appeared in print three months after the start of my residency at Sunnybrook in the University of Toronto's cardiology program. This brief article (10) may still hold the record for the quickest publication after the start of a residency, at least in Toronto.

I maintained my interest in coronary artery spasm as a cause of chest pain for several years. Initially, this condition attracted the attention of cardiologists working in the catheterization laboratory, with a variety of drugs being tested as possible treatments. However, by the 1980s, coronary artery spasm seemed to be forgotten, except in Japan, where studies have continued to be performed. I sometimes wonder how many women are still considered to be neurotic because they experience symptoms of chest pain related to spasm of their coronary arteries. I say women because the condition was rarely reported in men. There was never any explanation for this apparent gender difference. Perhaps it would have been studied in greater depth if more men had demonstrated spasm of their coronary arteries.

NINE

The Early Years at Sunnybrook

July 1, 1975 was my first day as a staff cardiologist at Sunnybrook. After four years of medical school and six more years of clinical and research training, I finally had a real job. However, my enthusiasm was tempered by the realization that I was now responsible for looking after sick patients with heart disease, even though I had less training in clinical cardiology than any other cardiologist in the university's teaching hospitals. On the other hand, I was moderately confident about my future career in research.

I became the sixth staff member of the Division of Cardiology. The division head was from a previous generation in which astute clinical knowledge and excellent skills in history-taking and physical examination were of paramount importance. My arrival meant that he no longer needed to take night- call and, being the newest kid on the block, I was placed on call every Friday night—for the next six years! However, I was so excited about my staff appointment that I gladly accepted this fate, at least for the first few years. My call schedule only improved when two more cardiologists were hired in 1982.

At this point, I think it would be of interest to explain how I survived as a clinical cardiologist. As I was far from confident about dealing with all aspects of cardiac disease, I quickly learned to seek advice from one or two of my colleagues whose knowledge I respected. My reading of electrocardiograms was sub-standard, so I took any tracing about which I was unsure to get a second opinion before writing the report. In this way, after several years, I became quite proficient in this task. The same approach was useful when I was faced with a complex case which I thought might benefit from the opinion of someone with more experience. By applying these principles to much of my clinical work, I was able to overcome the deficiencies in my cardiology training and become competent in the care of patients with heart disease.

I never considered myself to be lacking confidence. In my mind, I accepted that I might be an average clinical cardiologist, whereas I was going to be one of the top experts in hypertension in Canada. In this way, I acquired a thick skin if residents under my supervision ever questioned my competence, often because they saw me as a "researcher" and not a real doctor. I believe this is a hazard many researchers in medicine have to deal with when it comes to patient care.

I'm not sure how many of my colleagues remember the patients admitted to the Coronary Care Unit the first time they were on-call, but I certainly do. The second patient under my care was a transfer from a hospital in North Bay, a city in northern Ontario. He was seriously ill with a high fever, intermittent low blood pressure and a suspected underlying infection of unknown cause. When 36-year-old Mr. RM arrived, he was receiving two antibiotics and appeared quite ill. We stabilized his condition somewhat, mostly with intravenous fluids. Within a day, it was apparent that his blood pressure was fluctuating, from being very high to low, shock-like levels. We were unable to identify any infection, which was not surprising since he had already been started on antibiotics at the other hospital. He had no previous history of serious illness and had not seen a physician for years.

Given my training in hypertension, I soon focused on the wide swings in his blood pressure. The only condition I could think of was a pheochromocytoma, a (usually) benign tumour of the adrenal gland, which secretes hormones that stimulate the sympathetic nervous system. These hormones, norepinephrine and epinephrine, were the same ones I had been blocking with propranolol in my studies involving the brains of rabbits. The diagnosis of a pheochromocytoma was made by analyzing a 24-hour urine sample for the metabolites of norepinephrine. We obtained several 24-hour collections of urine and sent them out for analysis. The condition was so rare that only one lab in Toronto performed the assay.

While a pheochromocytoma was being excluded, the working diagnosis was still the much more common septicemia, in this case, an infection of unknown source which seemed to have spread to involve multiple organs in the body. To everyone's surprise, the urine test results came back highly positive. We now had a diagnosis, pheochromocytoma, which could be treated with a drug which blocks the sympathetic nervous system, phentolamine, the same intravenous drug we had used to prevent spasm of the coronary arteries. Mr. RM improved dramatically with the treatment. There had never been any infection.

After several weeks, the patient's condition was more stable and the pheochromocytoma was removed at surgery. I saw the patient a year later and he was doing well, without any further evidence of the tumour, something which was reassuring since a small percentage are malignant and do recur. A search of the medical literature turned up one or two similar cases of pheochromocytoma masquerading as septicemia. Since the condition was so rare, I decided to write it up as a case report, which was then published in the *Journal of the American Medical Association* (11). Case reports such as this can play an important role when it comes to diagnosing rare conditions. It is likely that several of the tens of thousands of doctors who read this medical journal would consider the possibility of a pheochromocytoma when confronted with a patient with similar clinical findings at some time in the future.

TEN

Larger is Not Always Better: The End of 70 mm Coronary Angiography

Instead of involving patients, one of my next studies examined the coronary angiograms which were being performed in our cardiac catheterization laboratory. The usual routine was to record a 35 mm cine-angiogram after the injection of contrast material into the coronary artery, which would then show if there were any blockages. The cine-angiogram was like a moving picture and the degree of obstruction in the artery was estimated by running the film back and forth while looking at the lesion on the screen. Each injection was also recorded on 70 mm film, with the pictures of the arteries appearing as photographs on plastic X-ray sheets. Multiple pictures were recorded for each lesion. The prevailing belief was that the lesions measured with calipers on the X-ray sheets provided a more accurate and consistent reading than was possible by estimating its size using the moving picture. I soon recognized that this was an opportunity to see if the 70 mm pictures were really better.

My task was to set up the experiment, while colleagues would estimate the extent of the lesions in the coronary arteries. I obtained a series of both 35 mm cine-angiograms and 70 mm X-rays on patients having a total of 52 lesions which were suitable for the study. Two radiologists and a cardiologist expert in coronary catheterization independently reported the blockages seen with the two techniques on two separate occasions, at least a week apart. The order of the 35 mm cine-angiogram and 70 mm x-rays was shuffled, so that the observers were not able to read the patients' two sets of films at the same time. Using this design, I was able to assess the variability in the readings between observers and within the same observer by comparing agreement among the observers in the readings for the 52 lesions and the within-observer agreement using the repeat readings.

From my perspective, this study was a true experiment, since I had no pre-conceived idea which method might be better. As it turned out, the overall agreement among the three expert observers was better with the visual estimate of the lesions using the moving cine-angiogram compared to the 70 mm x-rays, even though the clarity of the pictures was higher with the latter technique. Our findings did not prove that the 35 mm cine-angiogram was more accurate, since we could not assess the accuracy of either technique without measuring the actual lesions in the patients, which, of course, was not feasible. However, the results (12) were sufficiently impressive for the catheterization laboratory to abandon the 70 mm films, which simplified the entire procedure. Another group of researchers later reported similar findings and the use of 70 mm films for coronary angiography was soon discontinued everywhere.

I had now performed my second clinical trial, this time with X-rays and not a new drug. The principles were the same. Besides simplifying the catheterization procedure for physicians, the findings in this study ultimately reduced patients' exposure to unnecessary radiation, thus reducing the risk of developing cancer in the future.

During most of my career, I was never involved in only one research project at a time. There were two reasons for this. First, I was the only person in the Division of Cardiology who was doing independent research. Second, I needed to perform an unspecified number of studies in order to maintain my Ontario Heart Foundation scholarship. So, while I was collecting coronary angiograms for the above study, I also became interested in blood pressure and ageing.

ELEVEN

Studies in the Elderly

My arrival as a resident in Cardiology in 1974 coincided with the opening of a 420-bed long-term care facility for the ageing veterans at Sunnybrook. I soon recognized a new opportunity for research, this time in the field of geriatrics. In 1974, the prevailing belief was that blood pressure progressively increased with age until death or disability occurred. A book chapter (13) written by William Kannel, the Director of the Framingham Heart Study in the United States, included a figure which suggested that this belief might not be true. In the figure, systolic blood pressure readings tended to plateau at about age 60 in men and at 70 years in women. For unknown reasons, Dr. Kannel did not highlight these findings in the text. Perhaps he was uncertain of their validity.

Seeing an opportunity for a study, I sent my research nurse over to the veterans' wing to record blood pressure using a standardized protocol in as many of the ambulatory residents as possible, 90 percent of whom were male. A second part of the study was to record the blood pressure of all new admissions to the veterans' wing, with readings taken frequently during the first two weeks.

The results of our blood pressure survey (see Figure 2, opposite) confirmed what Dr. Kannel had reported. In 319 subjects, the systolic blood pressure (higher reading) continued to increase until age 65, and then remained at this same level. The diastolic blood pressure (lower reading) reached a maximum at age 55 years and then gradually decreased. We also noticed that the blood pressure of new admissions gradually decreased during the first two weeks after admission, becoming 10/3 mmHg lower than on the first day, which was enough of a difference to be important for patient management.

In this study, we had measured blood pressure with the patients sitting. However, we took this opportunity to examine the prevalence of postural hypotension (decrease in blood pressure upon standing) with increasing de-

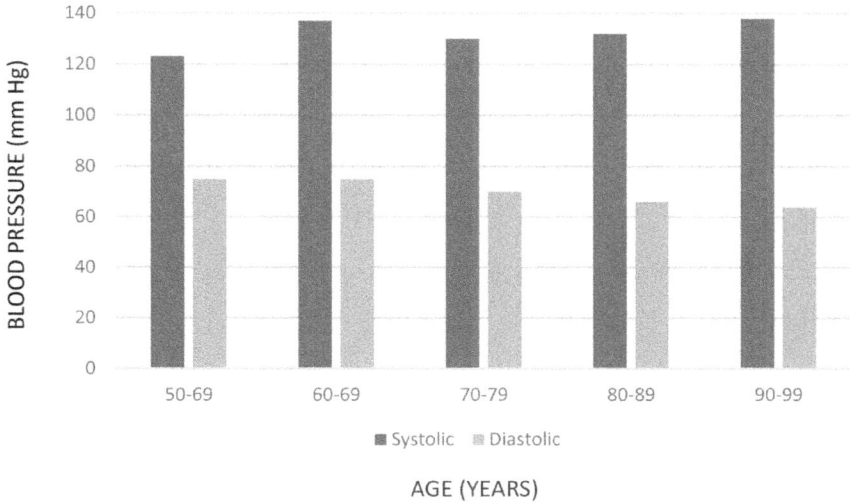

AGE (YEARS)
Number of Subjects: 50-69: 43 / 60-69: 56 / 70-79: 71 / 80-89: 136 / 90-99: 13

Figure 2. Mean systolic (dark columns) and diastolic (lighter columns) blood pressures of supine individuals in each decade between ages 50 and 99 years.

cades of age. The general belief was that postural decreases in blood pressure became greater in magnitude as one grew older. However, our data showed no such increase, with the changes in blood pressure upon standing in patients in their eighties being similar to those in their sixties.

We also found that 87 patients were receiving diuretic drugs (water pills) for a variety of reasons. These drugs were generally believed to cause postural hypotension. When we compared the patients who were on diuretics to those not taking these drugs, the occurrence and severity of postural hypotension were quite similar.

Several aspects of this study demonstrate my ability to recognize opportunities for performing clinical research. In the 1970s, the prevailing belief was that blood pressure increased with age. For many physicians, higher readings in the elderly were a "normal" occurrence and not a risk factor for experiencing heart disease and strokes in the future. By demonstrating that blood pressure did not always increase with ageing, our research opened the door for further studies. Subsequently, it became clear that the problem was not simply that the systolic blood pressure was higher in older age groups. As we grow older, our arteries lose their elasticity and become stiffer, which often leads to higher systolic and lower diastolic readings, starting at about age 60.

Thus, in an older age group, a blood pressure of 150/60 may be more harmful than a reading of 160/90 mmHg.

I submitted a manuscript describing what we had found in our studies to the *Canadian Medical Association Journal* for possible publication. In accordance with the usual routine, the paper was sent out for peer review, to be critically appraised by other researchers. In my case, one of the reviewers turned out to be Dr. David Sackett, who was the head of Clinical Epidemiology at McMaster University. I had never heard of him, but I knew he had reviewed the manuscript since he had signed his name to his review, which was quite unusual, since reviews are almost always anonymous. Dr. Sackett questioned several aspects of the study, but one of his comments took me by surprise. He asked how we knew that the decrease in blood pressure after admission to the veterans' wing was due to the patients now resting in a less stressful environment. Perhaps they were simply getting used to having the same person, the research nurse, record their blood pressure so frequently. I had not thought of this possibility.

We addressed the criticism by performing a series of blood pressure measurements over two weeks in veterans who were already residing in the institution. As Dr. Sackett had predicted, the blood pressure did fall with repeated measurements, although to a lesser extent than with the new admissions. We added these findings to our paper and it was accepted for publication (14).

I mention this encounter since it would have a lasting impact on my research career. Around this same time, I learned that Dr. Sackett and his colleagues had started offering a summer course in research methodology, which was being given at McMaster University two mornings a week during July and August. I signed up for the course, which involved being part of a group of four "students," all of whom were already in staff positions but were relatively new to clinical research. Without going into details of the course's content, I would summarize the learning experience as a lesson in how to perform studies using proper methodology without bias. Although Dr. Sackett was still several years away from introducing the term "evidence-based medicine," this concept was really what we had learned. It had a definite impact on my future studies by reinforcing my view that medical practice should be based primarily on scientific evidence and not on the opinion of "experts."

Attending the summer course in clinical epidemiology at McMaster also provided me with an opportunity to meet several others who were also interested in clinical trials and who would become my collaborators in later years.

The impetus to perform studies in the elderly was probably an outcome of my training at the Hammersmith. The British approach to educating a research trainee was to provide him/her with the opportunity to succeed. In many ways, it was either sink or swim, with no formal courses being offered on how to perform studies, analyze data or write manuscripts. In contrast, had I gone to train in the United States, I would have been required to attend post-graduate courses on various aspects of research, usually before performing any studies. Not everyone flourished under the British system. During my two years at the Hammersmith, I encountered several lost souls, who wondered how I had learned to do research. For me, it was a combination of having helpful colleagues, perseverance, a bit of luck and being able to recognize opportunities.

I continued further with my research interests in older patients who were taking diuretic medicines. There are two types of diuretics, those that remove excess water from the body and which are used to treat conditions such as heart failure, and those prescribed for hypertension. After seeing so many patients taking diuretics in my previous study, I wondered if doctors might be over-prescribing these drugs to this age group. Once again, I had a readily available population for a clinical study, residents of the veterans' wing at Sunnybrook Hospital. Since only a few of the veterans were women, I also enrolled female subjects from the Baycrest Home for the Aged, which was located not far from our institution.

In this study, we screened 885 residents and found that 276 were receiving diuretic drugs. Of these, 199 were excluded, mostly because there was good evidence that they were being treated for heart failure. I was left with 77 residents who did not have an obvious indication for taking this medication. Thirty-seven residents were receiving furosemide, which is usually used to treat heart failure, and the remaining 40 subjects were on thiazide diuretics used to treat hypertension. I was able to obtain matching placebo tablets for all the diuretic drugs. Subjects were then randomly allocated either to continue with their current diuretic medicines or take the matching placebo pills for the next 12 months. Only the pharmacists knew which patients were taking a placebo.

After 12 months, we found that the average blood pressure in the two groups was similar. Weight, a measure of the body's total water content, was also similar, despite removing the diuretic used to treat heart failure in 20 of the residents. To our surprise, 6 of the 17 patients who remained on the stronger furosemide diuretic developed heart failure during the 12 months of follow-up compared to only 2 of 20 who had this medication replaced with placebo (see Table 1 below). Hypertension developed in two of the subjects in the placebo group. We concluded that most of the residents had probably been treated with diuretics because they had swollen legs, likely due to spending most of the day sitting in a chair. These findings suggested that the elderly residents were often treated with diuretics when they didn't really need them, which is important to know, since older persons tend to take multiple medications. Taking drugs which are not necessary only increases the likelihood of a medication error. Moreover, diuretics were more likely to cause adverse side effects in the elderly, especially at the doses being administered to patients at that time.

Table 1. Reasons for withdrawal from the study in the two groups

Reasons for withdrawal (death)	Diuretic group	Placebo group
Heart failure	6 (1)	2 (1)
Hypertension	0	2
Dementia and malnutrition	1 (1)	0
Carcinoma	1 (1)	3 (3)
Respiratory disease	0	2 (2)
Stroke (normal BP)	0	1 (1)
Gastro-intestinal haemorrhage	0	1 (1)

Note: Fatal cases are noted in parentheses.

I was discouraged from performing more studies in this older age group because of the difficulties I encountered when trying to get the results of this randomized, placebo-controlled trial accepted for publication in a medical journal. Few studies of this complexity had ever been attempted in the elderly and the validity of the findings was never questioned. Nonetheless, several medical journals which often accepted studies of this type involving younger subjects were not interested in publishing one in which the participants had an average age of 82 years. Even though many editorials had been written about the importance of doing research in older people, when it came to actually publishing the studies, interest seemed to disappear. The article was eventually published in *Age and Ageing*. Despite this experience, I still had one more study to do in this older population.

As mentioned earlier, postural hypotension describes a decrease in blood pressure to abnormally low levels when a person stands after being seated or lying down. This phenomenon is associated with many conditions, including diabetes, Parkinson's disease and dehydration. It would therefore not be too surprising to find postural hypotension to be more common in older persons. The most common symptom related to the decrease in blood pressure is a feeling of faintness or even actual loss of consciousness. An association between low blood pressure and confusion had also been noted.

During my many hours of seeing older residents in our hospital's veterans' wing, I began to wonder how strong the relationship between confusion and hypotension actually was. Once again, the opportunity to satisfy my curiosity led me into new territory—the assessment of mental function.

My first task was to find collaborators who were experts in the evaluation of mental function, especially in the elderly. Pat Kearns was a clinical nurse specialist who was already working with the veterans. Ralph Shedletsky, a member of the hospital's Department of Psychology, had an interest in the mental assessment of older patients. The task for these two individuals was to help define the best population to study and to prepare questionnaires for the evaluation of mental function in this age group.

Once again, we recorded blood pressure readings in the veterans residing in the geriatric wing at Sunnybrook and found 12 extreme cases of postural hypotension. If anyone was going to suffer consequences from having a low blood pressure it would be these individuals. In this study, we used "mean" blood pressure (diastolic blood pressure plus one-third of the difference between systolic and diastolic blood pressure) for our assessment of the patient's blood pressure status. In the 12 residents with severe postural hypotension, the mean blood pressure decreased by 27 mmHg when they stood up after being supine, with the value on standing being only 65 mmHg, equivalent to a systolic/diastolic reading of 80/56 mmHg. We also selected another 10 residents who had similar characteristics to the postural hypotension group, without having a fall in blood pressure upon standing. These individuals were to be used as a control group.

At baseline, the average mental function test score in the 12 subjects with postural hypotension while supine was 42.3 and was unchanged (42.2) after three hours of being up and around. There was only a slight change in the score of the control subjects, from 49.9 while supine to 51.5 after walking around.

Mental function testing in the supine position was repeated in both groups after six months to see if there were any long-term effects of the low blood pressure. The mean test scores in both the postural hypotension group (40.4) and control groups (44.7) were both lower than before, with the controls exhibiting a greater difference than the residents with postural hypotension. We concluded (16) that chronically lower blood pressure readings upon standing in older persons did not appear to cause any deterioration in mental function. Moreover, the subjects of the study did not seem especially prone to feeling faint when standing, despite their low blood pressure. Of course, our sample size was quite small, but this limitation was offset by the severity of the postural hypotension and the absence of any dramatic changes after six months of follow-up. At the very least, the results of our study would encourage investigators to look for other causes of impaired mental function without having to consider low blood pressure as a contributing factor.

TWELVE

Nasal Decongestants and Blood Pressure

Almost everyone at one time or another has made a trip to their local pharmacy to seek out treatment for a head cold causing blocked nasal passages. The shelves are replete with various brands of decongestant nose drops, sprays and tablets, the latter containing ingredients which somehow find their way to the nose. The label on each package usually warns against using the product if you have high blood pressure. Being ever curious, I wondered about the evidence supporting these warnings, especially when most of the active ingredients had been on the market for years, before products such as these were routinely tested for safety.

One of the most common ingredients in nasal decongestants was phenylephrine (Neosynephrine). This product was selected because it tended to start working more rapidly compared to the others. If any of the drugs caused an increase in blood pressure, it would likely be one which was rapidly absorbed and fast-acting.

There was a reason for the concern that nasal decongestants might increase blood pressure. Phenylephrine is similar to norepinephrine, which, you may recall, was one of the substances secreted into the bloodstream which had caused the severe high blood pressure in my patient with the pheochromocytoma. Both substances will increase blood pressure within seconds after being administered intravenously. So, it should not be surprising that there might be concern about the effect of placing phenylephrine onto the nasal mucosa—the tissue lining the nasal passages—from where it would be rapidly absorbed.

Since there was little information from research studies on this topic, I saw an opportunity to assess the blood pressure responses to relatively high doses of phenylephrine nasal drops. There were two aspects to the experiment. First, higher than recommended doses of the phenylephrine nose drops would be administered in order to provoke an increase in blood pressure. Second, the experiments would first be performed in subjects with chronic nasal congestion and a normal blood pressure. If they did not exhibit an increase in blood pressure, then the drug would be administered to hypertensive patients.

On the test day, the subjects with chronic nasal congestion received increasing doses of phenylephrine nose drops at hourly intervals of 1.0 mg, 2.0 mg, 4.0 mg, 4.0 mg and 4.0 mg. The usual recommended dose of the phenylephrine nose drops was between 1.0 and 1.5 mg, taken every six hours. The subjects' blood pressure and heart rate were then monitored frequently until 120 minutes after the last dose. On the control group's day, a placebo solution identical to the phenylephrine, but without the active ingredient, was administered. The order of the two days was randomized and the investigators and subjects were unaware of contents of the nose drops.

The same study design was used for the 14 hypertensive patients who were receiving treatment with the beta-blocking drug metoprolol. The rationale for the experiment was that metoprolol's blockade of beta-receptors should predispose these patients to having a greater response to a drug such as phenylephrine, which stimulates alpha-receptors. Whereas beta-receptors in the wall of small arteries tends to cause them to dilate, stimulation of alpha-receptors in the same location tends to cause constriction. Hence, alpha- and beta-receptors provide opposing functions. Theoretically, blocking the beta-receptor with metoprolol would leave the alpha-receptors more susceptible to stimulation with phenylephrine, which would constrict the arteries, resulting in an increase in blood pressure.

As a precaution, a lower total dose of phenylephrine than with the normal subjects was administered, 0.5 mg, 1.0 mg, 2.0 mg and only a single dose of 4.0 mg, with blood pressure and heart rate again being monitored until 120 minutes after the last dose. The total amount of phenylephrine administered was 15 mg to the nasal congestion patients and 7.5 mg to the hypertensive patients on metoprolol, which was still 4 to 15 times the manufacturer's recommended dose. No significant changes in either blood pressure or heart rate were seen with either group. The highest average increase in systolic blood pressure after phenylephrine in the nasal congestion patients was only 5.0 mmHg, with most increases being less than 3.0 mmHg. Similar findings were seen in the experiments with the hypertensive patients and with both groups of control subjects. Since the small increases in blood pressure were similar on both the phenylephrine and control days, we concluded that using intranasal phenylephrine as directed was unlikely to cause a clinically important increase in blood pressure.

Although the sample size of both experimental groups was relatively small, we compensated for this limitation by administering phenylephrine at doses much higher than usually recommended. Keep in mind that this study was performed in 1982 and that it had been approved by the hospital's Ethics Review Board. I wonder if we would receive permission to conduct such a study today, given increased concerns about possible adverse effects form these higher doses.

The article which described our findings was published in the *Canadian Medical Association Journal* (17), since it was considered to be of general interest to a wide range of physicians.

After completing the experiments with phenylephrine nose drops, I decided to investigate further the possible interaction between this drug and beta-blockers used to treat hypertension. As mentioned earlier, there is a theoretical basis for the belief that taking a beta-blocker should predispose the user to greater increases in blood pressure when exposed to the alpha-receptor stimulant, phenylephrine. There had been little change in blood pressure when this drug was given by the intranasal route. My next study (18) was to see what would happen to blood pressure if phenylephrine was infused intravenously at increasing doses in patients receiving beta-blocker therapy.

The design of the study involved infusing phenylephrine on three separate occasions while patients were receiving either propranolol, metoprolol or a matching placebo. Propranolol was added to this experiment since it has an even greater beta-receptor blocking effect than metoprolol and would tend to make the blood pressure more sensitive to the effects of phenylephrine. Patients with a diagnosis of hypertension were treated for two weeks each with propranolol, metoprolol or matching placebo tablets, using a double-blind study design (neither investigators nor patients knew the identity of the tablets being taken during each two-week period).

Phenylephrine was given intravenously using an infusion pump which delivered the liquid in the syringe at a precise rate. The amount of phenylephrine administered was increased periodically at several pre-determined dosages until the systolic blood pressure had risen by at least 25 mmHg. Twelve hypertensive patients were enrolled in the study. The results (see Figure 3, next page) showed that the average dose of phenylephrine (mi-

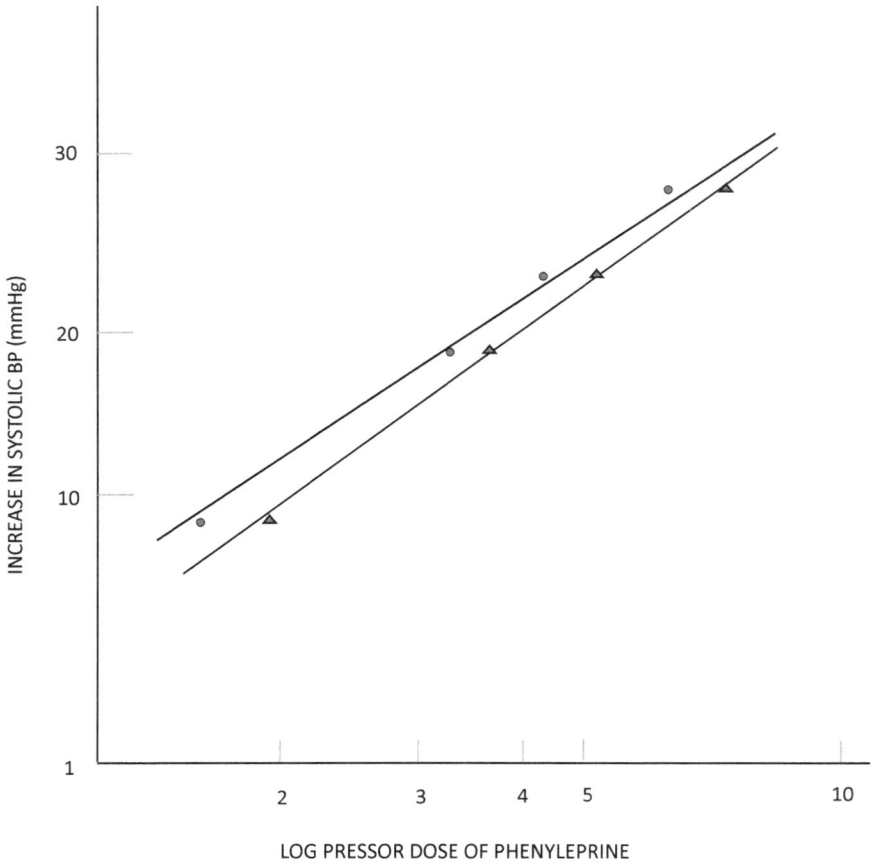

Figure 3. Increases in systolic BP are correlated with the log dose of phenylephrine (μ/kg) infused during propranolol and placebo therapy.

crograms/kg of body weight) required to increase the blood pressure by 25 mmHg was only slightly lower for propranolol (4.8) and metoprolol (4.7) than for the placebo (5.3), indicating that blocking the beta-receptors had little or no appreciable effect on the body's response to stimuli such as phenylephrine.

One aspect of this study which was somewhat unnerving was the heart rate response to the intravenous phenylephrine. At least one patient who was a marathon runner started the experiment with a heart rate in the low 50's. As his blood pressure tended to increase with the infusion of the phenyl-ephrine, the heart rate occasionally fell to the high 30's, due to the nervous system's (baroreceptor) reflex, which tries to keep the blood pressure from rising. Several other patients had their heart rate drop into the 40's. Nobody experienced any adverse effects.

These results confirmed the findings in our previous studies, showing that being on a beta-blocker would not likely increase the sensitivity of patients to recommended doses of nasal decongestants.

It is important to understand that these studies with nasal decongestants do not say that they are harmless or safe for everyone to use. What the findings do suggest is that the recommended doses should be safe for most patients who are concerned about experiencing an increase in blood pressure. Even those patients being treated with beta-blockers such as propranolol, metoprolol or atenolol may not be at increased risk of experiencing marked increases in blood pressure.

While on this subject, I have an anecdote to relate which was an almost fatal consequence of performing these research studies. I wasn't going to mention this episode, but my wife insisted that it be included. In doing so, I hope to erase any thoughts the reader might have about me having an inflated self-image. Nonetheless, it is still painful for me to relate one of the dumbest things I ever did, something which was almost fatal.

When doing research in medicine, it is possible to become identified as an expert on a specific topic. Experts can usually be found with a search of the medical literature, now made much easier by using Google or the Pub Med (Publications in Medicine) app. Such was the case with a number of my studies, including my work with phenylephrine. One day, about 15 years after the above experiments were published, I was asked by a law firm in Chicago to provide expert evidence in a case involving a lady who had possibly died from an overdose of phenylephrine nasal spray. I don't recall the details of the case, but an important aspect was the number of sprays one would get from a single container of phenylephrine nasal decongestant spray.

I was seeing patients in my office at the hospital, sitting in a small examining room, about 8 feet by 12 feet in size. I had purchased a container of phenylephrine nasal spray with the intention of determining how many sprays it would produce. When a patient failed to appear for a scheduled appointment, I closed the door and decided to conduct my experiment. I started squeezing the plastic bottle while counting the number of squeezes. After a while, I began to feel unwell and soon developed a pounding in my head and a throbbing sensation in my chest. I suddenly realized that I had been inhaling an overdose of phenylephrine. Since the spray hangs in the air for at least a few minutes, I had been breathing inside a cloud of phenyleph-rine. I quickly ran down the hall to the office of another cardiologist who was seeing patients and asked him to take my blood pressure. The systolic reading was over 300 mmHg, which is off the scale.

I asked him to run over to the Coronary Care Unit to get a vial of phen-tolamine, which is the antidote for phenylephrine. By the time he returned about 10 minutes later, I was starting to feel a little better. He took my blood pressure again and it was down to 260 mmHg. At least now it was back on the scale. The headache and throbbing in my chest were still present, but were a little less severe. We decided to hold off the intravenous phentolamine and my symptoms gradually disappeared. I had been very lucky. The only good part of the incident was that I now knew that the walls of my blood vessels must be strong and that I was unlikely ever to die of a brain hemorrhage.

The takeaway message from this incident is that anyone can make an (almost) fatal mistake, even doing something seemingly trivial. Obviously, I knew not to inhale the phenylephrine inside a small room, but I simply wasn't thinking at the time. Never spray aerosols in an enclosed space.

THIRTEEN

The Propranolol Withdrawal Reaction

In 1975, an article about the beta-blocking drug, propranolol, appeared in the *New England Journal of Medicine* (19), one of the most highly regarded medical journals in the world. In this instance, the drug was being used to treat angina, a discomfort in the chest experienced by patients who had at least partial blockage of the arteries supplying blood to the heart. The article reported on 6 of 20 patients (30 percent) who had a serious cardiac event within 14 days of abruptly discontinuing propranolol, which they had been taking as part of a study comparing this drug to a placebo. The other 14 patients did not have any serious problems. The authors called their finding the "beta-blocker withdrawal syndrome," which implied that the adverse event was the result of *abruptly* stopping the drug and that the same consequences would occur with all beta-blockers.

When I read the article, I interpreted the findings somewhat differently. The 20 patients were participating in this trial because they had serious heart disease with significant obstruction to blood flow in their coronary arteries due to the presence of cholesterol-containing plaques. To me, it seemed most likely that the patients had developed their complications not because of some adverse reaction to sudden discontinuation of propranolol, but because they were benefiting from taking it. Having propranolol stopped for 14 days resulted in a prolonged period of increased sympathetic activity which was associated with a faster heart rate and greater demand for oxygen on the part of the heart muscle. In the presence of severely narrowed arteries, the supply of blood to the muscle was reduced, making the patients susceptible to serious arrhythmias (abnormal heart rhythms) and/or a heart attack. The propranolol had been protecting them from these events. For unknown reasons, the authors did not say if the events occurred soon after the propranolol was discontinued or if some happened a week or more later. For the complications to be related to *abrupt* withdrawal, they should have occurred within days and not over a two-week period.

The findings in this article were contrary to the clinical experience at Sunnybrook Hospital where, for several years, propranolol had been routinely discontinued seven days before patients underwent coronary angiography. The rationale for stopping propranolol was based upon the belief that the drug depressed the strength of contraction of the heart muscle, making it more difficult to assess the ability of the heart to pump blood to the body. For this reason, it was thought best to stop propranolol before performing the test. Despite withdrawing it in every patient having coronary angiography at Sunnybrook, there had been hardly any withdrawal reactions, such as those reported in 6 of 20 patients in the *New England Journal of Medicine* article.

Before proceeding any further, I should explain that this medical journal was so highly regarded that most readers believed that anything published in its pages would almost certainly be true. Under these circumstances, it would have been difficult to obtain approval to initiate a new study to determine if a beta-blocker withdrawal reaction really existed. Fortunately, we already had data on the drug's sudden withdrawal in this patient population which provided me with an opportunity to perform two research studies.

For our first study (20), I reviewed the charts of the last 53 patients who had been receiving propranolol until it was discontinued for seven days before coronary angiography. There were two instances in which patients experienced cardiac complications. One patient had a transient worsening of his angina when taken off the beta-blocker, but underwent an uneventful cardiac catheterization after six days. The second patient experienced a fatal heart attack, but this occurred 10 days after the propranolol had been discontinued, far too long a time to call this a "withdrawal reaction" after "abrupt" discontinuation of therapy.

I should mention that the duration of propranolol's beneficial effect was relatively brief, such that the drug was usually taken four times a day in order to provide continuous 24-hour protection against angina. Thus, an abrupt withdrawal reaction should occur within two to three days and not up to two weeks. After three days, any cardiac event would more likely be due to the patient no longer taking the medication. Although our retrospective analysis of the 53 patients did not show any "abrupt" withdrawal reactions, it was not possible to make any definitive conclusions, since this was only an "observational" study. Perhaps it was simply by chance that the one patient out of 53 had a heart attack when off the drug after 10 days. Nonetheless, this ratio was strikingly different than the 6 of 20 patients reported in the article.

I decided it was now time to perform a second study, a proper randomized controlled trial (21). After the article in the *New England Journal of Medicine* had been published, it was no longer considered ethical to conduct a study involving abruptly stopping propranolol for a week because the risk to patients would be too high. Such a trial would involve randomly allocating patients with angina before cardiac catheterization either to propranolol or to a matching placebo tablet for seven days. Neither the patients nor their doctors would know whether propranolol or placebo was being taken. Instead, I chose a more feasible and ethically acceptable approach.

After the publication of the *New England Journal of Medicine* article, my colleagues who were doing the cardiac catheterizations began stopping propranolol therapy only two days before the procedure. Under these circumstances, I was able to assess the likelihood of a withdrawal reaction developing after propranolol was abruptly stopped by comparing the number of cardiac events during the 48 hours off the drug to the number of events which occurred during the 48 hours before withdrawal.

I decided that a sample size of 100 patients should be sufficient to obtain an answer, if the withdrawal reaction really did occur in 30 percent of patients, as reported in the published study. Upon completion of our study, two patients had experienced a non-fatal heart attack off propranolol and two patients had similar, non-fatal events during the 48 hours before withdrawal. Thus, our results had not confirmed the *New England Journal of Medicine* study's "abrupt withdrawal" theory. Although our study did not examine the effects of being off propranolol for seven days, the issue was no longer relevant, since there was no clinical reason to stop propranolol for more than 48 hours before cardiac catheterization. With propranolol being short-acting, 48 hours off the drug would be sufficient. Within a few years, it became standard practice to perform cardiac catheterization with the patient still receiving all their cardiac medications, including beta-blockers such as propranolol. By then, there was strong evidence that patients needed these medicines to prevent cardiac complications. I suspect that the "beta-blocker withdrawal syndrome" would never have become an issue if treatment decisions had been based on evidence from properly conducted research studies instead of on conjecture. The basis for withholding propranolol was always theoretical and illogical. By 1975, it should have been clear that beta-blockers were of great benefit to patients with coronary artery disease and that stopping this medication would have deleterious consequences for many individuals.

My involvement in the beta-blocker controversy was not over. After the two studies had been published, I received a call from the American pharmaceutical company which sold propranolol. During our conversation, I learned the full story behind the article in the *New England Journal of Medicine*. The sponsors of the study told me that the 20 patients had come from only one of several centres involved in a clinical trial in which propranolol had been stopped for 14 days. As I recall, there were more than 100 other participants in the study who did not experience the high rate of complications seen in the single centre. I was told that the cardiologists in the other centres were not especially trained in research and none of them was comfortable writing an article on the results of the entire study. Even though I had not been involved in the study, the company asked if I would be interested in writing such an article. Even in those days, this was an unusual request and for obvious reasons I declined the offer.

The story of beta-blocker withdrawal syndrome raises several issues related to medical ethics. An important feature of a clinical trial is to enroll sufficient patients in order to be reasonably certain that any positive or negative findings do not occur by chance. For example, in our study of 100 patients stopping propranolol, we did not anticipate that the event rate would be as low as 2 percent, since 30 percent of patients in the *New England Journal of Medicine* article had experienced an event when off propranolol. At the very least, we could conclude that any abrupt withdrawal reaction was likely to be infrequent. We could not be certain that it would never happen. With an event rate of 2 percent, it would have taken a study involving thousands of patients to make a definitive conclusion.

I imagine that the doctors at the centre where the event rate was 30 percent were faced with a dilemma: either to wait until the entire study was completed and see the overall results, or to publish their own findings because of a concern for patients, even though there was a possibility that the six events were a chance occurrence. The temptation to publish in the *New England Journal of Medicine* must have been very attractive.

Two decades later, a similar controversy occurred in Toronto when an investigator discovered that deferiprone, a drug used to treat patients with an excessive amount of iron in the liver, seemed to cause harmful adverse effects (22). Once again, the problem was noted in a relatively small number of patients enrolled in a multi-centre study. Reports suggested that the much larger sample of patients treated with the drug in the other centres had not experienced the same problem. Once again, the right to publish what was seen in a few patients in one centre before the entire study was completed became an issue. The ensuing debate generated considerable controversy in the scientific community. I am not sure if the issues were ever completely resolved, although a number of aspects specific to their study were addressed.

Thus, clinical trials are not always without controversy. The initial report on propranolol in the *New England Journal of Medicine* did not mention that the findings were coming from only one of several centres involved in the same clinical trial. Nonetheless, this report had a beneficial effect on the management of patients with coronary artery disease, with beta-blockers no longer being stopped routinely before catheterization was performed. In reality, there had never been much evidence to support this practice. I will leave it to the medical ethicists to deal with the issues surrounding the publication of the partial results of studies.

FOURTEEN

Stroke and the Heart

Nineteen seventy-four was a landmark year for Sunnybrook Hospital, as it was then called. Apart from my own arrival, a new 420-bed Veterans Wing had started accepting patients, the Emergency Department went from two rooms to being a major regional trauma centre and the McLaughlin Stroke Intensive Care Unit opened. Colonel Sam McLaughlin had been a pioneer in the automobile industry who converted his family's factory in Oshawa, Ontario from making carriages to automobiles in the early 1900s. Under a special deal with William Durant, who at the time was developing the Buick automobile, McLaughlin was able to build and sell the "McLaughlin," with some of the parts coming from the Buick factory in Michigan. By 1918, the car's name had changed to the McLaughlin-Buick, with Colonel McLaughlin establishing the Canadian division of General Motors with himself as president. Colonel McLaughlin's philanthropy included the creation of the world's first stroke intensive care unit at Sunnybrook Hospital, consisting of five beds with patients attached to cardiac monitors for the detection and documentation of any disturbances in the rhythm of the heart (cardiac arrhythmias).

Dr. John Norris was the director of the unit and he had recently recruited Dr. Vladimir Hachinski to help develop a research program in stroke. I was initially attracted to the Stroke Intensive Care Unit because of a possible association between stroke and cardiac arrhythmias. The presence of monitors in the unit provided an opportunity to study this relationship further. Moreover, one of the objectives of the unit was to provide an opportunity for further research in stroke and the heart.

About this time, a new, more specific enzyme for detecting cardiac damage began to be measured routinely in the hospital's laboratory. This enzyme, creatine kinase (CK), seemed to be present in many stroke patients who had no apparent cardiac abnormalities. In view of this finding, I decided to initiate a study together with doctors Norris and Hachinski. We proceeded to obtain blood samples from admissions to the stroke unit who had one of three diagnoses: stroke due to a blockage in an artery to the brain (cerebral infarction), bleeding into brain tissue (cerebral hemorrhage), and transient ischemic attack (transient blockage of blood flowing to the brain). A group of 64 patients who turned out not to have any of these diagnoses was included in the study as control subjects. In addition to the CK enzyme, we obtained a part of the CK, called the MB fraction, which was highly specific for damage to heart muscle. The patients were also monitored continuously for abnormalities in heart rhythm and with routine daily electrocardiograms.

After studying 224 patients, our suspicions were confirmed. Strokes could indeed cause diffuse damage to the heart muscle. Compared to the control subjects, significant increases in the cardiac enzymes, including CK-MB, were seen in all three types of strokes. Patients with higher levels of cardiac enzymes also had more abnormalities on the electrocardiogram and more cardiac arrhythmias on the monitor. Cardiac enzymes were highest in patients with cerebral hemorrhage. From these findings, we concluded that stroke, especially of the hemorrhagic type, may cause damage to the heart muscle (23).

The next task was to determine the mechanism by which an event in the brain was able to cause damage to the heart muscle.

In the experiments with rabbits, we had proposed that the effects of propranolol on the brain to lower blood pressure were likely mediated by the sympathetic nervous system, which is a network of nerves which exit from the brain, sending branches to various organs and to the arteries supplying blood to all parts of the body. The sympathetic nerves are partly responsible for the increase in blood pressure and heart rate when people are frightened or when performing exercise. When the sympathetic nervous system is activated, substances called neurotransmitters, such as norepinephrine and epinephrine, are released into the blood. Measurement of the concentrations of these substances is one way of assessing the activity of the sympathetic nervous system.

A suspicion that damage to the brain increased sympathetic activity led us to study patients admitted to the stroke unit to determine if stroke caused abnormally high blood levels of these neurotransmitters. In this study (24), we enrolled 74 patients with cerebral infarction, 18 with transient ischemic attacks and 33 non-stroke control subjects. The patients with either stroke or transient ischemic attacks had significantly higher levels of epinephrine and norepinephrine compared to the control subjects. Increases in blood pressure and heart rate were also significantly correlated with higher levels of norepinephrine.

As a result of these studies, it is not surprising to find evidence of heart muscle damage in patients admitted to hospital with a stroke, especially cerebral hemorrhage. Fortunately, such stroke-induced heart attack is relatively minor and does not affect the function of the heart. Rarely are further cardiac investigations required.

The admission of patients to the Stroke Intensive Care Unit subsequently identified another link between the heart and the brain. Sometimes patients presented to the unit with an obvious stroke, such as a paralysis of one side of the body, but when an electrocardiogram was taken, it was clear that a major heart attack had occurred. This latter relationship, which was relatively uncommon, later became the subject of a new finding. Some patients with a heart attack involving the anterior wall of the left ventricle (main pumping chamber of the heart) develop a blood clot on the inner surface of the damaged muscle which then travels to an artery in the brain, blocking the flow of blood and causing a stroke (cerebral infarction). These strokes are often quite severe.

As an aside, several years ago, when I was visiting a close relative in a stroke intensive care unit at a hospital in New York City (yes, there are now many such units), I was told by the resident that there may have been a heart attack at the same time as the transient ischemic attack that had led to the admission of my relative. Discharge had been delayed in order to obtain a cardiology consultation and various cardiac tests. The resident seemed unaware of the link between the brain and the heart. He left to see another patient before I could comment, but I did have an opportunity to speak with the nurses in the unit. I referred them to the publications of Myers, Norris and Hachinski which had identified the link between the brain and heart and which had elucidated the mechanisms involved. As I continued with my visit, a nurse approached me and started reciting from our 1981 article (24) on the sympathetic nervous system's role in causing cardiac abnormalities in stroke patients. Using the PubMed App on her phone, she had looked up my name and found the article. I was quite impressed by her initiative and she seemed pleased to have met such a famous researcher, or so I may have imagined. So, whenever you see a friend or relative in hospital and want to find out more about their illness, look it up on the Pub Med app on your mobile phone.

FIFTEEN

The Calcium Antagonist Story: From Clinical Trial to the Courtroom

The Clinical Trial

In the early 1980s, a new class of drugs called calcium antagonists became available for the treatment of hypertension. The drugs acted on the transport of calcium into the cells of muscle tissue lining the walls of small arteries called arterioles. These blood vessels were capable of dilating and contracting, depending on the status of these smooth muscle cells, especially in response to nervous stimulation. Contraction of the arterioles decreased the volume of blood they could carry, which led to an increase in blood pressure. Dilation did the opposite, which reduced blood pressure. Some of the calcium antagonist drugs, such as verapamil, also acted on the heart muscle to reduce contractility, which was useful in reducing the work of the heart. Patients with chronic blockages of the arteries supplying blood to the heart used verapamil to prevent chest pain (angina) when they exerted themselves.

The action of other calcium antagonists was directed more to the smooth muscle of the arteriolar wall, which made these drugs more useful for treating patients with hypertension. One such drug was called nifedipine (Adalat). Initially, medical researchers did not differentiate between verapamil and nifedipine, with their main interest for both drugs being in their use for treating angina. At the time, there were two ways of managing this condition, taking regular medication to prevent episodes of angina and taking rapidly acting therapy to abort an attack after the pain developed. Beta-blockers such as propranolol had become the primary treatment for the prevention of angina, whereas dissolving a small dose of nitroglycerine under the tongue was used to relieve angina after it had developed. There was also a topical ointment formulation of nitroglycerine which was applied to the skin several times a day in order to prevent angina. However, patients would develop tolerance to the nitroglycerine ointment, which resulted in a loss of its effectiveness.

Nifedipine was seen as being complementary to the beta-blockers, with the combination being more effective at preventing angina. The scientists at Bayer AG in Germany got the idea from the rapidly-acting nitroglycerine tablet that nifedipine might have greater efficacy if its onset of action was more rapid. As a result, nifedipine initially became available as a capsule containing the drug in a gelatinous substance which dissolved rapidly after it was ingested by the patient. The capsule formulation had both a rapid onset of action and also a relatively short duration of action, which necessitated the patient taking it every four to six hours. This feature was to become a double-edged sword.

Clinical trials suggested that the nifedipine capsule was effective for preventing angina, but investigators couldn't help noticing that it might also be good for treating hypertension. When nifedipine was given to patients with both angina and hypertension, there was a dramatic decrease in blood pressure. However, Bayer's primary interest was angina and the drug received approval for this condition, initially in Europe and by 1982 in Canada. Nonetheless, early on, nifedipine was also being used "off-label" (that is, for treatment of a condition for which it had not yet been approved) for the treatment of hypertension.

Although the nifedipine capsule did lower blood pressure, the rapid onset and offset of this effect was problematic. The ideal drug for treating hypertension should have a more prolonged duration of action, so that it could be taken once daily and still have a persistent beneficial effect over the entire 24 hours. Having a rapid onset of action was theoretically good for the rapid relief of angina, but not for hypertension. Abrupt decreases in blood pressure could cause some patients to become lightheaded or even to faint. The Bayer Company recognized this problem and proceeded to perform clinical studies on a new tablet formulation of nifedipine, called Adalat PA ("PA" standing for "prolonged action"), which was absorbed more slowly and had a longer duration of action, enabling the drug to be taken twice daily.

In, 1983 Dr. Frans Leenen and I were invited to a meeting on nifedipine in Scheveningen, Holland, which is a suburb of Den Haag. We stayed at a wonderful old hotel called the Kurhaus, which had been the headquarters of the Gestapo in World War ll. Dr. Leenen had come to work at the Toronto Western Hospital after receiving his clinical and research training in cardiology, clinical pharmacology and hypertension in Holland. Since our research backgrounds were almost identical, we had become interested in collaborating in studies involving new treatments for hypertension. Today, company-sponsored meetings such as this one are often frowned upon, but in 1983 they were a useful opportunity for investigators such as Dr. Leenen and me to learn more about new drugs which might not yet have appeared in Canada.

The audience consisted of about 50 researchers, mostly from Europe, some of whom had already been using Adalat PA in treating their patients. During the presentations over the next two days, it was evident that Adalat PA should be a much better formulation for treating hypertension than the rapidly-acting capsule. After ingestion, its antihypertensive effect was gradual in onset and persisted for 8 to 12 hours. We left Holland convinced that Canadian doctors should be using Adalat PA instead of the capsule for treating their hypertensive patients. However, the Canadian subsidiary of Bayer had been told by head office that they were to only market the capsule, since the company intended to sell another calcium antagonist, nitrendipine, which was thought to be similar to Adalat PA, in both the United States and Canada.

The Canadian affiliate very much wanted Dr. Leenen and me to perform a research study in hypertension, but we insisted on using Adalat PA instead of waiting for nitrendipine to become available. Our persistence paid off. Thus, we became the first investigators in North America to do a clinical trial using Adalat PA.

Unlike angina, there were already many drugs available for the treatment of hypertension. Since nifedipine was the new kid on the block, we were limited to studying it only in patients who had a persistently high blood pressure, despite being on two other drugs, a diuretic and a beta-blocker. The study was designed to compare Adalat PA to another drug, hydralazine, which at the time was being used in combination with the other two medications.

Today, such a clinical trial would generally involve multiple hospitals with 100 to 200 patients being enrolled. But in 1983–4, we were able obtain evidence to support using Adalat PA by studying its effects in only 23 patients. Patients were randomly allocated to receive each drug for nine weeks with the doctors and nurses performing the study unaware of the order of the two treatments. Nifedipine lowered blood pressure significantly more than hydralazine and was well tolerated by the patients. The results of this relatively small study (25) were quite promising.

I subsequently did a second study (26) which examined the relative concentrations of the nifedipine capsule and tablet in the blood and their effect on blood pressure in patients with hypertension. Such a study may only require a few patients to demonstrate significant results, especially when the capsule and tablet were so different in how they lowered blood pressure. All six subjects received both formulations of nifedipine, in random order on different days. Two 10 mg nifedipine capsules caused a dramatic fall in blood pressure within 45 minutes (see Table 2, opposite), with the blood pressure going from an average of 177/98 at baseline to 117/75 mmHg. In contrast, a single 20 mg Adalat PA tablet produced a gradual decrease in blood pressure from 179/102 to 145/87 mmHg over a four-hour period.

Since the capsule had already been identified as a useful treatment for lowering blood pressure rapidly in patients with severe hypertension, the marked fall in blood pressure in our subjects was not surprising. As you will see in a later section, high blood pressure readings, especially in the elderly, are often due to a "white coat effect," which is an anxiety-induced response to having blood pressure recorded in an office setting. In many of these individuals who might not even have been hypertensive, the administration of the nifedipine capsule could easily have reduced blood pressure to very low levels. The resulting sudden reduction in the flow of blood to vital organs could cause a heart attack or stroke.

Adalat PA was soon available for the treatment of hypertension in Canada. As for American patients, the approval of nitrendipine, which was supposed to replace the nifedipine capsule, was delayed for years. American physicians continued prescribing the more rapidly acting capsule until a long-acting, once-daily formulation of nifedipine became available.

Today, nifedipine and other calcium antagonist drugs are widely used for the treatment of hypertension. Adalat XL and another long-acting calcium antagonist, amlodipine, are especially useful in patients whose blood pressure is difficult to control. The shorter-acting formulations of nifedipine are now only of historical interest. A unique aspect of this class of drugs is that the higher the dose, the more the blood pressure falls. Other treatments for hypertension tend to exert most of their effect at lower doses, whereas, with calcium antagonists, the logarithmic value of the administered dose or the amount of drug in the blood is directly proportional to decrease in blood pressure. The main dose-limiting factor is side effects, the most common being swollen legs, which usually develop with prolonged periods of sitting or standing.

Table 2. Supine blood pressure, heart rate, and plasma nifedipine concentration after administration of nifedipine capsules or a nifedipine tablet

	Hours								
	0	0.25	0.5	0.75	1	2	4	6	8
Capsules[a]									
BP[b]	177/98	154/86	123/78	117/75	124/75	136/78	144/82	143/84	161/91
HR[c]	65	69	71	68	67	67	64	66	68
Tablet[d]									
BP	179/102	181/99	162/96	155/91	151/92	157/88	145/87	149/86	164/93
HR	64	66	66	68	65	65	66	69	62
Capsules (N)[e]	0	39	163	223	192	108	58	32	24
Tablet (N)	0	1	13	27	25	33	38	33	23

[a]Two 10 mg nifedipine capsules. [b]BP, supine blood pressure (mm Hg). [c]HR, heart rate (beats/min). [d]One 20 mg nifedipine capsule. [e]N, plasma nifedipine concentration.

Meeting at the Health Protection Branch

Until recently, I would forever have been known more for my legal exploits than for anything I did during my career in research, at least according to Google. This section is more about the perils of doing research than it is about any one study. It all began in December 1994, when I was invited to attend a meeting of the Health Protection Branch of the Canadian government in Ottawa. This agency is the Canadian equivalent of the American Food and Drug Administration. One of its tasks is to regulate the use of pharmaceutical products in Canada. The issue for discussion at the meeting was quite simple. It related to the wording of the product monograph for a new, once-daily formulation of nifedipine, Adalat XL, and how doctors should switch over their patients from the older, twice-daily Adalat PA to once-a-day Adalat XL. The meeting lasted only a few minutes and Adalat XL was soon approved.

Nine months later, in September 1995, I was invited back to the Health Protection Branch, this time to participate in an ad hoc cardiovascular advisory committee. Other attendees included my colleague Dr. Leenen, another specialist in hypertension and a research cardiologist. The Acting Director of the Cardiovascular Division of the Health Protection Branch was the chair of the meeting and several other members of the division also attended, including Dr. Michelle Brill-Edwards.

Besides the study done with Dr. Leenen using Adalat PA, I had been the chair of a committee of the Canadian Hypertension Society that recommended diuretics and beta-blockers as the preferred therapy for the treatment of hypertension, with drugs such as nifedipine to be prescribed only if these two drugs did not prove effective. I had also published a study (27) in 1988 which had raised concerns about the use of the nifedipine capsule in patients with angina. At the time, it was my opinion that Adalat PA should replace the capsule for every purpose, except for the emergency treatment of patients with very high blood pressure levels, where a rapidly acting drug might be advantageous. Indeed, by 1995, Adalat PA and Adalat XL had virtually replaced the nifedipine capsule in Canada. As for Dr. Leenen, I assumed that he had been invited because of his previous research and clinical experience with calcium antagonists, the class of antihypertensive drugs we had been asked to review.

The meeting of the four-member committee lasted four hours. We reviewed two recent articles (28, 29) from the United States which had raised concerns about the use of nifedipine, primarily the capsule, which was still in widespread use in that country. The articles had suggested that nifedipine might be causing cardiac complications and should no longer be prescribed to patients. There was general agreement among the four of us that the problem was with the capsule formulation and that there was little evidence for nifedipine itself being harmful. We recommended that long-acting, once-daily Adalat XL be used, that other drugs such as diuretics and beta-blockers should be prescribed first for treating hypertension before considering the addition of a calcium antagonist, and that diltiazem or verapamil should be prescribed to patients with both angina and hypertension. Our recommendations were consistent with the Canadian Hypertension Society's guidelines for the treatment of hypertension.

Three months later, on January 23, 1996, the Health Protection Branch sent a letter to all Canadian physicians outlining the possible concerns which had been raised about calcium antagonists. The letter ended with a series of recommendations for their use in patients with hypertension and heart disease. As I recall, the letter warned against the use of the nifedipine capsule for the treatment of hypertension. We were not shown an advance copy of the letter and did not participate in drafting it.

Enter *the fifth estate*

Meanwhile, the Canadian Broadcasting Corporation (CBC) program, *the fifth estate*, a weekly investigative journalism program similar to *60 Minutes* that is still on the air, got involved. Its staff had been alerted to a potential "cover-up" at the Health Protection Branch by Dr. Brill-Edwards, who had been present at the advisory board meeting. My only previous interaction with her had occurred when I was director of the clinical pharmacology residency training program at the University of Toronto about 10 years before. She had been successful in applying for a two-year residency position at the Hospital for Sick Children, under the supervision of Dr. Stuart MacLeod. Other than approve her appointment, I had very little interaction with her following our initial meeting. I only found out about her involvement with *the fifth estate* when the program was aired. Subsequently, I was told that she had been passed over for a promotion at the Health Protection Branch soon after the Advisory Board meeting and had resigned her position.

In December, three months after the Advisory Board had met, I was contacted by someone from *the fifth estate,* asking if I would agree to be interviewed about the use of calcium channel blockers in the treatment of hypertension. Until this time, I had often spoken with members of the media and had frequently been on television and radio. In preparation for the interview, I sent the CBC copies of articles related to the calcium-channel blocker controversy. I also included a copy of the Canadian Hypertension Society's guidelines (30) for the treatment of hypertension, which recommended diuretics and beta-blockers as preferred therapy and mentioned that I had chaired the guidelines committee.

Although the interview was supposed to last for only one hour, the television crew remained in my office for four hours. The interviewer, Trish Wood, was quite aggressive with her questions. She seemed to want me to talk about the dangers of nifedipine, but I mostly confined my comments to the scientific issues and to the Canadian recommendations which placed nifedipine as a third- or fourth-line drug. An unusual aspect of the interview was that the producer, Nicholas Regush, remained outside of my office until the session was over. He then introduced himself to me and said that we had met once before, which, at first, I did not recall. Subsequently, I was reminded that he had previously interviewed me and another hypertension expert in Montreal, Dr. Jacques de Champlain. I don't recall the details, but I do remember that Mr. Regush proceeded to write an article in the Montreal newspaper where he worked which suggested to readers that high blood pressure was being over-diagnosed and that patients may not need to take their medications. At the time, Dr. de Champlain was furious, since great efforts were being made by the Heart Foundation and other organizations to get patients to treat their hypertension in order to reduce the risk of strokes and heart attacks. You will shortly see why I have mentioned this incident.

After the CBC staff left my office, I was satisfied with how the interview had gone, although it hadn't been my most pleasant experience with a television host. I thought we had discussed the most important issues and that I had been given an opportunity to present the Canadian perspective on the drug treatment of hypertension and the appropriate role of the calcium antagonists. However, I was somewhat puzzled by the belated presence of the producer at the end of the interview.

It would not take long before I learned more about what was happening. I soon discovered that *the fifth estate* was interviewing some of my colleagues who got the impression that the program was now more interested in the relationship between academic physicians and the pharmaceutical industry. However, I could not recall anything in my own interview which would have fit in with this topic. I became even more curious when I received a telephone call from the CBC a week before the program was to go on the air. They asked if I would be willing to do a second interview. As I had already spent four hours answering numerous questions, I turned down their request. Also, by then, I had heard about other interviews from colleagues and was beginning to suspect that the program might have a hidden agenda, beyond just the treatment of hypertension.

On February 27, 1996 the program appeared on the CBC national television network. To say I was shocked by the first few words spoken would be a gross understatement. The interviewer, Trish Wood, led off by saying "nifedipine, taken every day in the country by hundreds of thousands of people," may have caused a huge number of deaths. Dr. Brill-Edwards then appeared saying "the numbers (of deaths) are off the scale… We're talking about thousands, tens of thousands, maybe more than that, worldwide certainly."

Subsequently, Dr. Curt Furberg from North Carolina, who had written one of the two articles suggesting calcium antagonists might be harmful, repeated Dr. Brill-Edwards' point that "we're probably talking tens of thousands of patients dying as a result of patient taking these pills [the nifedipine capsule]." Two excerpts from my interview followed. I said that there was some circumstantial evidence that the short-acting capsule might be harmful, but that there was no evidence that the longer-acting nifedipine tablet might also be harmful. I then described the differences between the nifedipine capsule and the long-acting nifedipine-XL, which had now replaced the tablet and capsule, with the latter's use by then being extremely rare in Canada. (I should note that the same was not true in the United States, where the nifedipine capsule was still widely prescribed and where the two articles warning about the nifedipine capsule had been published. However, the program was addressing a Canadian audience and not Americans.)

Dr. Leenen also was treated unfairly in the program. They distorted his comments and questioned his judgement and integrity. We were both very much victims of a biased and malicious representation of what had transpired at the Health Protection Branch meeting.

The program sent a clear message to its viewers that the ad hoc medical advisory committee had covered up a major scandal involving tens of thousands of deaths and that I had promoted the use of nifedipine. There was no mention of my support for the Canadian guidelines at the meeting, nor was anything said about my position that the calcium antagonists should only be used after other drugs had failed to control the hypertension. They also did not mention that I was the only person at the advisory board meeting who had clearly stated that the nifedipine capsule should be removed from the market, since it might be harmful, whereas there was no evidence implicating the longer-acting versions of the drug.

Moreover, the program did not report that a month earlier, on January 25, the Food and Drug Administration in Washington had convened an open meeting to hear different viewpoints on the calcium antagonist debate. The FDA concluded that the drugs were safe if used according to their product monographs. Nothing was said about the nifedipine capsule being responsible for tens of thousands of deaths.

When I returned to the hospital the morning after seeing *the fifth estate* program, I was extremely concerned about how its content had been received by my colleagues and by the hospital administration. Relief came quickly. By 9 a.m. my division head had been called into the president's office to discuss what had transpired. He was told that two members of the board of trustees had already called to ask "Who is this Dr. Myers and what has he been up to?" Dr. Brian Gilbert, who was well respected in the hospital, replied that I was a responsible physician and excellent researcher and that the content of the program had been extremely biased and grossly exaggerated. I was never asked to appear before the president, nor did I ever hear a word of criticism from the administration or from any board member. I had been at Sunnybrook for more than two decades and most of the medical staff and administration knew me. They recognized that my reputation had been maligned and I had become a victim of the program. I subsequently wrote an article in the *Canadian Medical Association Journal* in which I described the events surrounding my encounter with *the fifth estate* (31).

To the Courtroom

The support of my colleagues was most welcome, but it did not alleviate the emotional upset which lingered long after the program was shown. I could not stop wondering what the many patients I had seen during my years at Sunnybrook now thought of me. The clear message from the program was that I had supported a drug which was killing tens of thousands of people. I felt that I had to do something and decided to seek a legal opinion to see if there were grounds for a libel suit. My intention was to pressure the CBC into offering me an apology, which would be shown on the television network and reported in the newspapers. I never anticipated going to court.

It turned out that my daughter's close friend was the daughter of Julian Porter, the lawyer who "wrote the book on libel in Canada." When I met with him, he made it clear that I had been a victim of libel, but he added that the CBC would never apologize. If I were to go any further, I should be prepared to see the action through until its conclusion.

Our second meeting was at a restaurant in the early evening. After a thorough discussion of the case and a tasty meal, Porter said he would call a taxi for a ride home. Instead, he accepted my offer of a lift. We continued talking until I was about two blocks from his house. He stopped in mid-sentence and blurted out the words, "How did you know where I lived?" He had never told me his address. It was then that I revealed the friendship between our two daughters and told him that I had driven my own daughter to his house on several occasions.

By then, I had decided to proceed, at least to the first step, which was to prepare a statement of claim which described the libel. A series of surprises followed. No, the CBC did not offer to apologize. Their response was to ask that the court disqualify Porter from my case since his wife had been the editor of a book published by one of the defendants, Nicholas Regush, who, you will recall, was the guest producer hired by the CBC to supervise the program.

I was now without legal counsel, but at least I had been given his opinion—I had a strong case for libel. Porter recommended another law firm and they referred me to one of their lawyers who had recently gone into practice on his own. Chris Ashby was an expert in libel and had worked for several years as an in-house lawyer for another Canadian television network. His hourly fee was also lower than my first choice, who was highly sought-after because of his expertise and reputation. Legal costs would certainly be an important factor for me to consider if the action were to progress further.

There was yet another mountain which I would have to climb, if I were to succeed. The lawyer for the CBC was Ian Binnie, a senior partner at McCarthy Tetrault, the major national law firm which represented the CBC. Mr. Binnie was recognized as one of the foremost courtroom litigation lawyers in Canada. Chris Ashby (you will see later on why we are now on a first-name basis) was not overly optimistic about our chances. However, as soon as we started working on the case, Mr. Binnie was appointed to the Supreme Court of Canada. We had clearly been given a break. The trial, by itself, could easily be the subject of an entire book. Instead, I will do my best to present the highlights.

Early on, we had a small but important victory. Chris was an expert in the media and knew that what had been shown on the program was only small part of what would have been recorded in my office. It seems that film crews like to run their cameras as much as possible, even when there is no interview taking place. Chris proceeded to ask the court to have the CBC provide us with the "outtakes," which included everything recorded on the day of the interview. Despite vigorous opposition from the CBC's lawyers, the judge agreed to our request. From the outtakes, we were able to see derogatory comments such as "let's get the (obscenity)," "let's see if we can trick him into saying …" and other incriminating statements on how to make me give the answers they wanted to hear. There was also no shortage of obscene remarks directed toward me.

The trial took place in November 1999, and lasted for more than five weeks. I took my place sitting beside Chris who had asked me to take notes, since he was a sole practitioner and did not have an assistant. My wife, Patty, sat a few rows back, among the other attendees. Across the courtroom sat four or five lawyers representing the CBC and its staff. It was a David and Goliath scenario.

I was cross-examined on the witness stand for more than a week. Justice Denise Bellamy had only been on the bench for two years and was very careful not to reveal her thoughts during the exchanges between the witnesses and lawyers. In response to numerous leading questions from Mark Freiman, the principal lawyer for the CBC, I continued to quote the Canadian guidelines for the treatment of hypertension, which considered calcium antagonists to be useful third-or fourth-line medications for treating hypertension. After a while, he seemed to become quite frustrated with my reluctance to agree with any of his introductory statements without adding some qualification. It was my way of avoiding any trap I might fall into.

One highlight occurred during Patty's testimony. Chris had put her on the stand to tell the court how upsetting the program had been for the two of us. This part of the cross-examination had been given over to a relatively junior lawyer, David Leonard, who was assisting Mr. Freiman in the case. He began by asking Patty a few harmless questions about herself, but he did not ask about her occupation. He then proceeded to ask what she had thought about my "promotion" of calcium antagonists during the program (which was untrue). Patty became visibly upset and responded that if I had promoted these drugs, she would have divorced me. After all, she was a marketing manager for a pharmaceutical company which sold a drug for the treatment of hypertension which was not a calcium antagonist and was a direct competitor of nifedipine. After describing her work, she went on to say that I had always refused to give lectures involving her product or do any research with it because I considered this to be a conflict of interest. Mr. Leonard, looking quite flummoxed, hesitated and then said, "No further questions, Your Honour." It was only a small victory early in week 2, but it made Patty feel as if she had done her part. Mr. Leonard's appearance in the trial occurred early in his career. This experience was probably a minor setback for him, since he went on to become the Chief Executive Officer of McCarthy Tetrault.

Once the CBC defendants began taking the witness stand, the case took on more serious overtones as we were now on the defensive. Chances of success appeared especially poor every Friday afternoon, when the CBC's position seemed to be strengthening, only to be put into perspective on the following Monday. On other days, we had to deal with misleading testimony from the defendants. One morning, Dr. Brill-Edwards claimed that I had spoken favourably about the nifedipine capsule nine times during the advisory board meeting. I knew this to be untrue. When Chris asked her to point out the sentences in the transcripts of the Advisory Board meeting where I had given this support, she asked for a recess. Returning an hour later, she softly said that she could not find any examples, but that she was certain I had said this.

Throughout the proceedings, Chris showed great skill in uncovering the hidden agenda of Mr. Regush and his co-workers. He was able to show how they had set out to portray me as a supporter of nifedipine, regardless of how I answered their questions. Mr. Regush was an especially good witness for us, in that he was forced to admit that the story for the program had been prepared in advance, even before any interviews had taken place.

A seemingly innocuous question from Chris was to make a long-lasting impression on the CBC. The program claimed that nifedipine was responsible for tens of thousands of deaths and yet the CBC waited for several months before telling Canadians about these deaths. David Studer, who as executive producer of the program had hired Mr. Regush took the stand. Before his testimony, I encouraged Chris to ask him why the story had not been on the CBC's newscasts, if there had actually been so many deaths from taking nifedipine. Chris, being a cautious lawyer, was reluctant to do this, since he had not asked this question during discovery, when lawyers get an opportunity to meet and question witnesses from the other side. Since I often listen to the news on the CBC, I was certain the answer would be that the story had not been reported on the CBC's newscasts. When Chris had almost finished his cross-examination, I began pulling on his gown, imploring him to ask the question. By then, he had come to trust my memory of events and, reluctantly, he asked if the story had been reported on the CBC news. Mr. Studer paused for what seemed like an eternity and then replied "No." We had scored a major victory. It was clear that the CBC did not really believe that the drug had killed thousands of people. As the famous journalist, H.L Mencken once facetiously said, "Never let the truth get in the way of a good story."

After Chris asked this question, the CBC has always included newsworthy content from *the fifth estate* on the CBC national news a few days before the program goes on air. More than 20 years later, the question has still maintained its impact.

There were many more exchanges between witnesses and lawyers, but one I clearly recall was a comment made by Mr. Regush during his testimony. He said he did not believe in taking drugs for hypertension. Instead, he preferred more "natural" therapies. Sadly, he would experience a fatal heart attack several years later related to his poorly controlled hypertension. He was only 58 years old.

As the time in court was coming to an end, we thought we had done okay, but the judge's poker face gave no indication of the verdict. Overall, I was extremely pleased with Chris' performance, first in obtaining the outtakes from the film crew, then thoroughly examining the details of the defendants' written notes and finally in an expert cross-examination of each witness. Patty and I knew that if we lost, we would need to pay the legal costs of the CBC, probably several million dollars, likely leading us into bankruptcy.

The verdict came several months later. The judge had found the CBC guilty of libel and had awarded me $200,000 plus costs. The victory was especially welcome, considering the consequences of losing. The trial had other milestones. It was the most important trial for both Justice Bellamy and Chris Ashby up to that time and it was the last court appearance for Mark Freiman, who then went on to become Assistant Deputy Minister in the Office of the Attorney-General.

My ordeal was not yet over. The following year, the CBC proceeded to the Ontario Court of Appeal in front of a three-judge panel, including Chief

Justice Roy McMurtry. The CBC took one and a half days to present their arguments, with their lawyers frequently being interrupted by the judges. Chris had prepared three to four hours of material for his presentation, but after 30 minutes, he sat down. I had to wait until the judges had left the courtroom before getting an explanation for his change in plans. Chris, quite calmly, said that the judges were listening very politely to what he was saying and, unlike the session with the CBC lawyers, they were not interrupting him and asked no questions. "Why go on any further?" he said. "They were clearly on our side."

Chris had been right. Not only did the judges reject the appeal, but they said Justice Bellamy had only made one error—she had not given me a sufficiently high award—so they almost doubled the amount. A further appeal to the Supreme Court of Canada, which was evaluated by Chief Justice Beverly McLachlin herself, was also rejected. The original verdict had been upheld. If you are interested in reading more about the trial, you should read an article by Dr. George Carruthers (32) written after the appeals were rejected.

The Aftermath of the Trial

Not only was this case the most important victory in Chris Ashby's career up to that time, but it also brought him other rewards. I knew that he had been divorced for several years. A friend had told me that her boss, who was a senior executive, was a wonderful person who somehow had managed to escape marriage. I convinced Chris (you can see now why he is not Mr. Ashby to me) to meet her and they ended up getting married. Mr. and Mrs. Ashby have remained our close friends ever since.

I realize that these events have little to do with medical research, other than demonstrating the potential pitfalls of acquiring a reputation as an expert in a particular field. However, I cannot resist adding a brief anecdote, this time involving a patient. You will soon see the connection.

Around the time of the appeal to the Supreme Court of Canada, I was on-call for the Coronary Care Unit at the hospital. After retiring for the night, I received a telephone call from the resident in the unit saying that a patient had gone into heart failure again and was not expected to survive. I was reluctant to accept such a verdict on the telephone, so I drove to the hospital and found an older gentleman gasping for air and quite moribund. I noticed that one drug had not yet been tried and added it to his treatment. Even I was surprised at how quickly he improved, becoming less short of breath and more alert. What made this patient even more special was his family. I went out to the visitors' waiting room and who should I find but Justice Bellamy, who had presided over my trial, and her husband, who was the son of the patient.

I still remember the judge's words when she stood as I entered the room: "You stood every day when I entered the courtroom, now it's my turn to stand for you." After updating them on the condition of the patient, we had a pleasant chat, without delving too deeply into the trial. I believe her father-in-law lived another six or seven years. Every time his wife accompanied him on visits to see his cardiologist at Sunnybrook, she also came by my office to say hello. I had found another way to thank the judge.

It would be no surprise if I said that my experience with *the fifth estate* had a major impact on my relationship with the media. Until 1996, I had likely spoken with reporters about hypertension once or twice a month. Paradoxically, the CBC was probably my best partner. Although I was obviously reluctant to speak with anyone in the media during the court proceedings, I still had some interesting interactions. As part of my hospital practice, I looked after several senior executives working at the CBC. The most prominent one actually encouraged me to continue with the libel suit. He/she was certainly no fan of *the fifth estate*. The others did not seem to be bothered by an "enemy" looking after them. In fact, I got the impression that the program was not very popular among others working in News and Public Affairs. Even before the final appeal was denied, I once again began receiving requests from reporters at the CBC for comments on various items related to hypertension. At first, I declined to respond, but then I started giving interviews on non-controversial subjects after first reminding the reporters about my history with the CBC. Strange, but each caller said there was no problem with me being interviewed. It seems that any problems related to *the fifth estate* did not extend to other departments of the News and Public Affairs division of the CBC.

SIXTEEN

Preventing Heart Attacks with Aspirin

Next, I would like to describe a study which was performed at six teaching hospitals affiliated with McMaster University (Hamilton), the University of Western Ontario (London) and at Sunnybrook Hospital. Many readers will have seen advertisements on the television extoling the benefits of Aspirin in preventing heart attacks. Not too long ago, the use of Aspirin was mostly restricted to pain relief, such as treating simple headaches. However, a Canadian research study contributed new knowledge which led to an expansion of the indications for taking Aspirin.

The main part of the study was a comparison of Aspirin versus placebo in patients with unstable angina (chest pain at rest due to plaques obstructing the coronary arteries) who were at risk of experiencing a heart attack. The study originated at McMaster University with Dr. John Cairns as the principal investigator. My participation occurred by chance. The original plan was to have cardiologists at the Toronto General Hospital recruit patients in the Toronto area for the study. However, the cardiologist at this centre encountered several obstacles which made it impossible for him to join the study. I was subsequently told that members of the Division of Cardiology would not agree to have their patients tied up in a single study for the three years it would take for recruitment and follow-up. However, I suspect there was another reason. The Toronto General Hospital had a long history, going back to 1821, and in the 1980s was probably the primary centre for cardiology research and training in English Canada. McMaster was a relatively new university and this was one of the first clinical trials from its cardiology division. Cardiologists at the other Toronto hospitals speculated that the reason for declining participation was that the study did not originate from the Toronto General.

As I mentioned earlier, I had already developed a connection with McMaster and also knew Dr. Cairns from 1969, when we had both done our pediatric internship at the Montreal Children's Hospital. Dr. Sackett, my mentor in clinical trials, was also involved in the study. So, I should not have been surprised to find out that Sunnybrook was now being considered as a replacement for the Toronto General Hospital. By this time, patients in London and Hamilton were already being enrolled in the trial. Keep in mind that I was only a co-investigator. Nonetheless, my participation would provide me with an opportunity to apply some of my newly acquired skills.

My first task was to obtain approval of the study and its patient consent form from Sunnybrook's Research Ethics Board. In doing so, I had the benefit of seeing the submissions which had already been approved by the boards at the hospitals in Hamilton and London. One item in the consent forms caught my attention: "gastrointestinal symptoms" and an "upset stomach" were mentioned as possible side-effects of the Aspirin, which the subjects had a 50 percent chance of taking. By the time, multiple reports in the media had associated these symptoms with Aspirin, although they were usually considered to be mostly a nuisance and rarely serious. I decided to omit any mention of gastrointestinal upset from the Sunnybrook consent form, but did include more specific side-effects such as gastrointestinal bleeding, abdominal discomfort, vomiting, diarrhea and constipation. When I told my colleagues in Hamilton and London about my plans, they said it was too late to make any changes to their own hospitals' consent forms.

After receiving approval to conduct the study at Sunnybrook with our version of the consent form, we enrolled 156 patients, bringing the total number of participants in the study to 555. The final results of the study were astounding (see figure). There was a 71 percent reduction in cardiac death and death from any cause in the Aspirin group compared to the event rate in the patients randomly allocated to the placebo group. Also, there was a 51 percent reduction cardiac death and non-fatal heart attack in those randomized to receive Aspirin. Rarely is a treatment ever this effective.

Only 16 of the Sunnybrook patients (10 percent) withdrew from the study because of side effects compared to 110 patients (28 percent) at the hospitals in Hamilton and London. These were mostly minor gastrointestinal side effects, which occurred in 25 patients at Sunnybrook and in 175 at the other hospitals. Of the 200 patients who had reported minor side effects, upon completion of the study we found that only 56 percent were actually taking Aspirin, indicating that something else was responsible for these symptoms. From our perspective, the obvious reason for the much lower rate of minor

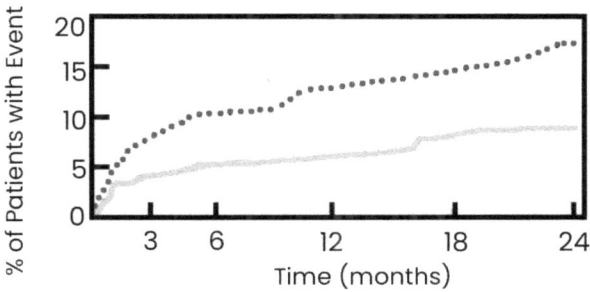

Figure 4. Occurrence of cardiac death or nonfatal myocardial Infarction (MI) in the Aspirin (solid grey line) and No Aspirin (dotted line) groups.

The graph is a life-table depiction of the cumulative risk and time of first occurrence of an outcome event, according to Aspirin allocation. Numbers of patients at risk are as follows:
Aspirin total at 0: 263. At 3 months: 174. At 12 months: 137. At 18 months: 107. At 24 months: 73.
Non-Aspirin total at 0: 274. At 3 months: 180. At 12 months: 144. At 18 months: 115. At 24 months: 80.

side effects at Sunnybrook leading to withdrawal from the study was the absence of any mention of gastrointestinal upset in the consent form. Had the withdrawals from the study at Sunnybrook been similar to that of the other hospitals, the overall rate would probably have been closer to 70 percent, which would have made the overall findings of little or no value. Too many subjects would not have completed the two-year follow-up period, making it impossible to evaluate possible benefits of Aspirin therapy versus the drug's possible adverse effects.

Once again, I realized that this chance observation was, in itself, quite important. I proceeded to publish a separate article (33) using data from this study, entitled "The consent form as a possible cause of side-effects," documenting the impact that omitting gastrointestinal upset from the consent form had on the study.

During the ensuing years, specialists in medical ethics have periodically contacted me to ask about the role the consent form played in this study and how it was possible to omit gastrointestinal side effects. My response has been that many people in 1985 would have known about the association between Aspirin and gastrointestinal upset. The letter to the family doctors in Hamilton and London, which described the study, had also mentioned this side effect as a possibility, something to watch for. It was therefore not surprising that most of the decisions for patients to withdraw from the study were made by their family doctors and not by the cardiologists in the study. By the time the patients had returned for follow-up, they had already stopped their study medication. Once again, I had recognized an opportunity to report a seemingly insignificant finding, which had a major impact on the success of what was to become a landmark scientific publication. After the publication of this study and another article (34, 35) in the *New England Journal of Medicine*, patients with coronary artery disease began to be routinely treated with Aspirin to prevent heart attacks.

Considering my previous interest in dose-response studies, I feel obliged to comment on the dose of Aspirin used in our study. Patients were given a 325 mg tablet four times a day, for a total of 1,300 mg. Aspirin was so effective that even this huge dose was still associated with more benefit than harm from side effects. Today, the dose is as low as 81 mg. Not very many drugs have ever been as beneficial to patients as Aspirin was in our study, even when given at 16 times the optimal dose.

SEVENTEEN

The Cardiovascular Effects of Caffeine

Caffeine and Cardiac Arrhythmias

Many of us have experienced palpitations after drinking too much coffee. In keeping with my inclination to question the obvious, I wondered if drinking coffee really did cause disturbances in the rhythm of the heart (cardiac arrhythmias) that would be experienced as palpitations. Always interested in new opportunities for research, I thought about designing a study to see if caffeine actually caused cardiac arrhythmias. I could only find one brief report (36) which suggested such an association, but the number of subjects in this study was quite small and the results were not statistically significant.

As often happened, I was busy with other projects, so this opportunity was kept in reserve, until one day when I heard about Dr. Harold Grice and a granting agency in Washington which provided funds for research on caffeine. Dr. Grice was the Scientific Officer of the International Life Sciences Institute (ILSI) grants committee which was mostly comprised of scientists employed by companies whose products contained caffeine, such as cola beverages and coffee. I contacted Dr. Grice at his home in Ottawa to say that I was thinking of doing a study to see if caffeine caused cardiac arrhythmias. He seemed quite interested in my proposal, perhaps because he also liked the idea of having the committee support research in Canada.

From here on, I will mostly use coffee and caffeine interchangeably. I should make it clear that the culprit is not really the coffee bean, but the caffeine which it contains. The average 200 ml cup of coffee may contain anywhere from 100–200 mg of caffeine, depending on how it is brewed.

I submitted an application to ILSI with the protocol designed to expect a positive outcome, that is, to show that caffeine did indeed cause cardiac arrhythmias. I didn't take into account the committee's preference to see that caffeine did NOT cause any cardiac problems. After all, their salaries depended on the sale of caffeine-containing beverages. To my surprise, not only did the members recommend that ILSI fund the study, but they gave me the full amount I had requested. Dr. Grice had been a good advocate for my research.

Once again, I was fortunate to have a population close at hand who could serve as subjects. Unlike the rapid turnover of cardiac patients in hospital today, in the 1980s patients admitted with a typical heart attack spent several days in the Coronary Care Unit followed by a week or more on the cardiology ward. During this time, the hospital provided only decaffeinated coffee, which contained a negligible amount of caffeine. One reason for this practice may have been a concern that cardiac arrhythmias, which were commonly seen following a heart attack, would become worse after the ingestion of caffeine. Alternatively, they may have wanted the patients to be resting quietly and not responding to any stimulation from ingesting caffeine.

By then, we knew that regular consumption of caffeine tended to cause tolerance, in that the brain and other organs in the body adjusted to habitual exposure to caffeine. As a consequence, if people drank coffee at work Monday to Friday, but none on the weekend, by Sunday, they might be subject to having caffeine withdrawal symptoms, such as headaches. Also, others who had not recently consumed caffeine, would tend to be more sensitive to any possible adverse effects, including cardiac arrhythmias, when they returned to drinking coffee.

For the study, I recruited 70 patients admitted with a heart attack who had not consumed any caffeine during the previous 5 to 10 days in hospital. Each subject was given 300 mg of caffeine or an identical placebo powder, each dissolved in 250 ml of decaffeinated coffee, with the drinks being given in random order on different days. The investigators were unaware of the day when caffeine was being administered. If caffeine did cause cardiac arrhythmias, they might be more likely to occur in someone who had recently experienced a heart attack, because the electrical system of the heart is more unstable in the presence of recent damage to cardiac tissue. In fact, coronary care units had initially been created to detect and treat cardiac arrhythmias, which were a common cause of death during the first week after a heart attack. The study was approved by Sunnybrook's Ethics Research Board, since there was no actual evidence that caffeine would be harmful to the participants in the study.

After these caffeine-free subjects were given the equivalent of two to three cups of coffee at one time, the rhythm of the heart was monitored continuously to detect any possible increase in cardiac arrhythmias.

We were somewhat surprised that this amount of caffeine did not adversely affect the heart, with the number of abnormal heart-beats being similar on both the caffeine and placebo days. We even measured blood levels of caffeine to show that a relatively high concentration was present during the entire four hours of monitoring the heart rhythm. Not only was there no change in the occurrence of cardiac arrhythmias with caffeine, but the heart rate did not increase. This aspect of caffeine's effect will be discussed shortly.

We concluded (37) that drinking the equivalent of two to three cups of coffee after abstaining from caffeine for several days did not cause any adverse effects in patients at increased susceptibility to experiencing cardiac arrhythmias. Needless to say, the Scientific Committee of ILSI was very pleased with the findings. I was surprised.

Not content with stopping here, I decided to repeat the study using a higher dose of caffeine and a longer period of monitoring of the heart rhythm. Using a similar study design, I administered 300 mg of caffeine or a placebo, each dissolved in decaffeinated coffee, to 35 heart attack patients under the same conditions as in our first study. Four hours later, each subject received an additional 150 mg of caffeine or placebo. The heart rhythm was monitored continuously for eight hours. Since the initial dose of caffeine was the same as in the first study, we combined these subjects with the other group of 70 patients in order to examine the heart rhythm during the first four hours. Even with a total number of 105 individuals, we still did not see any increase in cardiac arrhythmias. Furthermore, there was no increase in the frequency or severity of cardiac arrhythmias after the higher dose of caffeine 450 mg compared to placebo in the 35 subjects during eight hours of monitoring. These findings (38) confirmed the initial conclusion that ingestion of the equivalent of three to four cups of coffee over a relatively short period of time did not cause cardiac arrhythmias.

What about the palpitations frequently associated with drinking coffee? Could they represent an increase in the normal heart rate, considering that caffeine is a stimulant which increases the activity of the sympathetic nervous system? If this was the cause, we should have seen an increase in both blood pressure and heart rate. Starting 30 minutes after the ingestion of caffeine, there was a small increase in blood pressure, which persisted during the remainder of the study period. However, we were quite surprised to see that the heart rate after caffeine not only did not rise, but actually decreased. We thought we had made an original observation. However, upon searching the medical literature, we discovered a publication from 1968 (39) which had reported similar findings in healthy normal subjects. Thereafter, I was always reluctant to claim that any discovery was "original. (See the later section on ambulatory blood pressure and caffeine ingestion for a detailed explanation for the decrease in heart rate.) However, our findings could also explain the sensation of palpitations which many coffee drinkers experienced. Caffeine also increases sensory awareness, including our subjective feelings. The slower heart rate coupled with an increased awareness of the heart beating could be interpreted as an abnormal cardiac rhythm.

Around this time, a colleague sent me an article from *Discover* magazine entitled "If coffee isn't bad for you it should be." I think these words succinctly describe the attitude many people have to coffee drinking.

Several years later, I wrote another article on coffee and cardiac arrhythmias, which was published in a prestigious American journal, the *Annals of Internal Medicine* (40). This time I reviewed all of the existing literature on the subject, concluding that moderate ingestion of caffeine/coffee did not increase the frequency or severity of ventricular arrhythmias in normal persons, in patients with ischemic heart disease or in those with serious pre-existing ventricular arrhythmias. Subsequent studies have not contradicted these findings.

Caffeine and Coronary Artery Disease

Coffee has also been associated with a variety of illnesses, including heart attacks. Having investigated a possible link between coffee/caffeine and cardiac arrhythmias, I next turned my attention to coffee and heart attacks. In this instance, I collaborated with Dr. Anthony Basinski, who was an expert in performing meta-analyses, which involves combining the data from multiple studies of the same condition to obtain more definitive findings in a much larger number of subjects than present in the individual studies.

We decided to look at the incidence of heart attack or death from coronary artery disease in people with varying amounts of coffee consumption. Following an extensive search of the literature, we found 11 studies which had examined these events in persons who regularly consumed from one cup or less up to six or more cups of coffee a day. The chance of having a coronary heart disease event (heart attack) was arbitrarily set at 1 in 100 for persons consuming one cup of coffee or less per day (see figure). For those persons consuming up to six cups of coffee daily, the risk of having a heart attack was

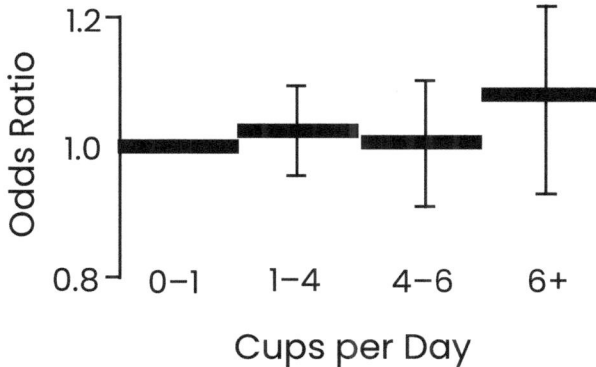

Figure 5. Odds ratio for coronary heart disease events for all studies at each range of coffee intake relative to coffee intake of 1 cup or less per day.

still only 1 in 100. Even the ingestion of more than six cups a day was associated with only a 10 percent increase in cardiac events, which was not of any clinical or statistical significance (41).

At the time, our findings were not widely accepted, since they disagreed with the prevailing belief that coffee consumption was indeed bad for the heart. However, smoking turned out to be a confounding factor. There was a strong association in the population between coffee drinking and cigarette smoking. Since cigarettes were a well-known cause of coronary artery disease, coffee tended to get blamed for an increase in cardiac deaths, because many heavy smokers also drank a lot of coffee. In our analysis, we had taken into consideration the smoking status of the subjects. Subsequent meta-analyses, which also controlled for cigarette smoking, have shown that caffeine, by itself, does not increase the risk of heart attack, thus confirming our own conclusions.

Effects of Caffeine on Blood Pressure

Given my interest in hypertension, it should not come as a surprise that I next took the opportunity to examine more closely the relationship between coffee/caffeine and blood pressure. As before, I reviewed the scientific literature on the subject of caffeine and blood pressure. As of 1987, there had been 17 studies which examined this topic, nine of which were small and had fewer than 50 subjects. Others contained from 500 to 80,000 persons. The overall findings (42) were that caffeine did not cause any *persistent* increase in blood pressure. Individuals who do not regularly consume caffeine may experience slight increases in blood pressure when they drink a strong cup of coffee, but tolerance develops quite rapidly with continued exposure and blood pressure returns to normal after several days.

Although these conclusions were based on a considerable amount of data, not all of the studies were in agreement. Several smaller, positive studies were overshadowed by the largest studies, which did not show any persistent effect of caffeine on blood pressure, beyond the brief, slight increase seen before the development of tolerance.

Several years later, I decided to use a new approach to evaluating an individual's blood pressure—24-hour ambulatory blood pressure monitoring—to demonstrate the increase in blood pressure in caffeine-naïve subjects, the development of tolerance and the return to the previous level of blood pressure after the cessation of caffeine exposure (43). Ambulatory blood pressure monitoring provided an opportunity to obtain meaningful results by studying a much smaller population, since this method recorded blood pressure and heart rate automatically every 15 minutes for 24 hours without any human involvement, which could be a source of bias. This procedure involves the subject wearing a small device attached to a blood pressure cuff during usual daily activities and produces 50 to 70 readings over the next 24 hours.

When 200 mg of caffeine was given at 9 a.m. and again at 1 p.m., the average blood pressure increased from baseline reading on day 3 of 124/76 to 127/79 mmHg on day 6, the first day caffeine was consumed. This small but statistically significant increase in blood pressure was accompanied by a significant decrease in heart rate of three beats per minute. By the third day of daily caffeine administration, the blood pressure had returned to baseline. Heart rate also showed a transient decrease, which was the body's response to the increase in blood pressure. These changes in blood pressure confirmed the conclusions which had been made in our earlier experiments involving patients with heart attacks. Ingestion of moderate to large doses of caffeine on blood pressure in caffeine-naïve persons causes only a small, transient increase in blood pressure, with tolerance soon developing.

Why does caffeine decrease heart rate? For those who are interested, the most likely explanation involves the response of the baroreceptor reflexes of the human central nervous system. I previously mentioned what happened to the heart rate in the study when phenylephrine was infused intravenously. In those experiments, the heart rate decreased, similar to what occurred in

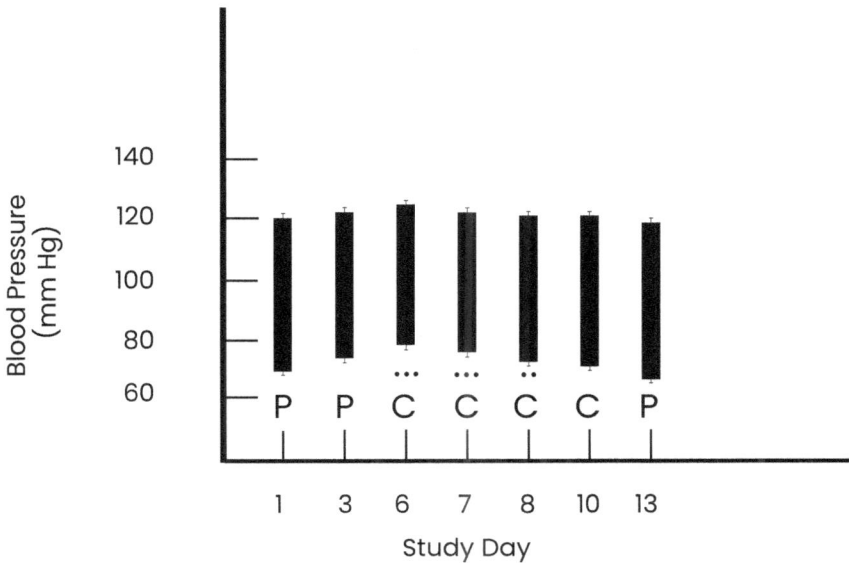

Figure 6. Illustrates Changes in Blood Pressure During Ingestion of Caffeine (C) and Placebo (P). Levels of Significance vs. Baseline,. Day 3: •••P<.001; ••P<.01

our caffeine experiments in heart attack patients. Both phenylephrine and caffeine tend to increase blood pressure, but there is an opposing reflex in the brain (the baroreceptor reflex) which tends to offset this increase, by enhancing the activity of other (parasympathetic) nerves, which slow the heart rate. For this reason, heart rate and blood pressure do not always both increase in response to stimuli. The fall in heart rate is the body's compensatory response to the rise in blood pressure.

When it comes to blood pressure, the message for coffee drinkers is that you should consume your coffee daily, regardless of how much you ingest. Otherwise, if you miss a day, you might get a caffeine withdrawal headache and be subject to a small increase in blood pressure when you have your next cup.

There are reasons why caffeine has received so much attention in research studies. The most obvious one is the popularity of coffee in the general population. From the perspective of scientific research, caffeine is a naturally occurring drug which is not subject to the usual restrictions of other manufactured chemicals. Anyone can do a study with caffeine, provided that ethical issues are satisfactorily addressed. As I discovered with my own articles, medical journals seemed interested in publishing studies whose results are either positive or negative. Even though the findings showed that caffeine was not harmful, all of my articles were readily accepted by some of the top scientific journals. Although there have been numerous studies published in the 25 years since my last article involving caffeine was published, the results of the experiments which I have described are still considered to be valid.

EIGHTEEN

The Cardiovascular Effects of Cigarette Smoking

As previously mentioned, coffee drinking and cigarette smoking are behaviours often seen in the same individuals. Thus, having been attracted to the cardiovascular effects of caffeine/coffee, it was logical for my attention to turn next to cigarettes. In the 1980s, patients admitted to hospital could still smoke, at first in their rooms and later in the decade in a separate room set aside for this purpose. However, patients admitted to the Coronary Care Unit for heart attacks or prolonged chest pain (angina), could not smoke until they were discharged to the ward. Previous studies had reported conflicting results when patients with coronary artery disease had their heart rhythm monitored while smoking cigarettes during various activities. Once again, I had a captive population of admissions to the Coronary Care Unit who were smokers before admission and who were anxious to return to smoking as soon as possible.

I saw another opportunity for a study by providing them with six cigarettes, one every 30 minutes during which time their blood pressure and heart rhythm were monitored and blood samples taken. Some of the 52 subjects were still in the Coronary Care Unit and the others who were on the ward had not smoked since the previous day. The patients were randomly allocated to four hours of observation after smoking on one day and simulated smoking, sucking on a straw, on another day. Continuous monitoring of the heart rhythm over four hours showed no increase in cardiac arrhythmias during and after smoking the six cigarettes compared to the control day. The first cigarette caused a transient, small but significant increase in blood pressure of 4/3 mmHg and in heart rate of 3 beats/minute. Thereafter the blood pressure and heart rate returned to baseline levels without any further changes. Sympathetic nervous system activity appeared to increase with blood levels of norepinephrine and epinephrine both showing a significant increase on the smoking day. Thus, involvement of the sympathetic nervous system precluded any decrease in heart rate in response to the rise in blood pressure, as had occurred in the caffeine studies.

Thus, we did not confirm our hypothesis that cigarette smoking in patients with active coronary artery disease would cause an increase in cardiac arrhythmias. Now came the hard part—to get a study published which showed that smoking did *not* cause something harmful. Even though we had designed a randomized, placebo-controlled, clinical trial and had executed it carefully, the first few cardiology journals rejected the submitted manuscript, despite the reviewers having given it a high rating. Finally, I sent the manuscript to *Chest*, which was the most highly rated journal for the publication of articles on lung disease. In the letter to the editor (which routinely accompanies submitted manuscripts), I pleaded that I would say anything he wanted to indicate that smoking was harmful, if he would consider publishing our paper. To my surprise, the manuscript was accepted (44) and it is probably still one of the few published studies which does not implicate smoking as being a health hazard.

Thus, my studies on cardiac arrhythmias came to an end. Even though they had been somewhat tangential to my other research, I thought it was important to know if some of the common activities of daily life might have potentially serious adverse effects. Part of the attraction had been my interest in using clinical trials to address questions which would be of interest to a wider audience, beyond the medical profession. Had the results been positive, showing coffee or cigarettes to be harmful in the situations that I studied, then I likely would have persisted with more studies. Instead, I was on to other areas of cardiology.

NINETEEN

Performing Unnecessary Tests after a Heart Attack

There are considerable differences in the amount of money that different countries spend on health care. Among developed countries, Canada allocates a relatively high percentage of GDP to keeping its population healthy. However, the money spent on health care in all countries, including Canada, is relatively small in comparison to such spending in the United States. Americans spend 50 percent more per capita on health care than most western countries and yet their life expectancy is only average, more recently even in decline. Private health care in the U.S. is frequently motivated by profit, which may be one reason why American patients are more likely to undergo investigations of unproven benefit. Canada's proximity to the United States makes our health care system vulnerable to being influenced in both good and bad ways by our southern neighbours. However, most Canadians, when told that they should have a specific investigation, usually don't question the advice, since health care plans in this country generally do not encourage a profit motive.

As a cardiologist who began practice in the 1970s, I had an opportunity to see the number of diagnostic tests increase dramatically as new technologies were introduced. For example, the exercise test for possible coronary artery disease went from walking up and down two wooden steps, the Master's two-step test, to walking on a treadmill at increasing speeds and inclines. Other advances included the detection of cardiac arrhythmias with 24-hour monitoring of the electrocardiogram and evaluation of heart damage by ultrasound or using radioisotope scanning devices. The rationale for performing the additional tests was to identify abnormalities such as signs of ischemia (decreased flow of blood to the heart) on the exercise test, evidence of potentially serious arrhythmias on the 24-hour electrocardiogram, or to learn the extent of damage to the pumping chamber of the heart, which could lead to a poor prognosis after a heart attack.

In the late 1980s it had become routine practice for patients admitted to Sunnybrook Hospital with a heart attack to have all of these tests prior to being discharged home. Their popularity was based upon the belief that the additional information would enable cardiologists to identify patients who were at increased risk of experiencing another cardiovascular event or complication related to their heart attack. However, having the results of the tests available did not necessarily mean that they were useful predictors of outcome. They might even be harmful, such as having a patient exercise on a treadmill so soon after a heart attack or receiving high amounts of radiation from the radioisotope used in the heart scan. Being curious, I wondered if these tests were of any benefit, which prompted me to design a study to determine if their routine use in patients who had experienced a heart attack improved the cardiologist's ability to predict the risk of a recurrent cardiac event during the next 12 months

One hundred and forty-seven patients who had been admitted to the Coronary Care Unit with a heart attack were enrolled into the study. All patients had the usual routine blood tests, electrocardiograms and at least one chest x-ray. Patients were also followed daily, including with a physical examination, in order to detect any complications while in hospital. Participants in the study also had a treadmill exercise test, a 24-hour tape recording of their electrocardiogram to detect any arrhythmias and a nuclear scan of the heart to determine the extent of damage that the heart attack might have caused to the left ventricle, the main pumping chamber of the heart. The results of these three tests were withheld from the patient's own cardiologist and the resident physicians who were also looking after the patient.

At the time of the patients' discharge from hospital, their staff cardiologist and two other cardiologists were independently shown a summary of their findings in hospital, including the electrocardiogram, chest x-ray, results of routine blood tests and any abnormalities on the physical examination, such as the presence of heart failure. The cardiologists were then asked to predict the chances of the patient experiencing another heart attack or death from a cardiac cause within the next 12 months using a scale from 0 to 10, with 0 being no event and 10 being very certain that an event would occur. The cardiologists were then given the results of the treadmill exercise test, 24-hour ECG monitoring and assessment of the heart function and were again asked to make a second prediction, based on the previous information and the results of the patient's additional tests.

Patient's own cardiologist

Second cardiologist

Third cardiologist

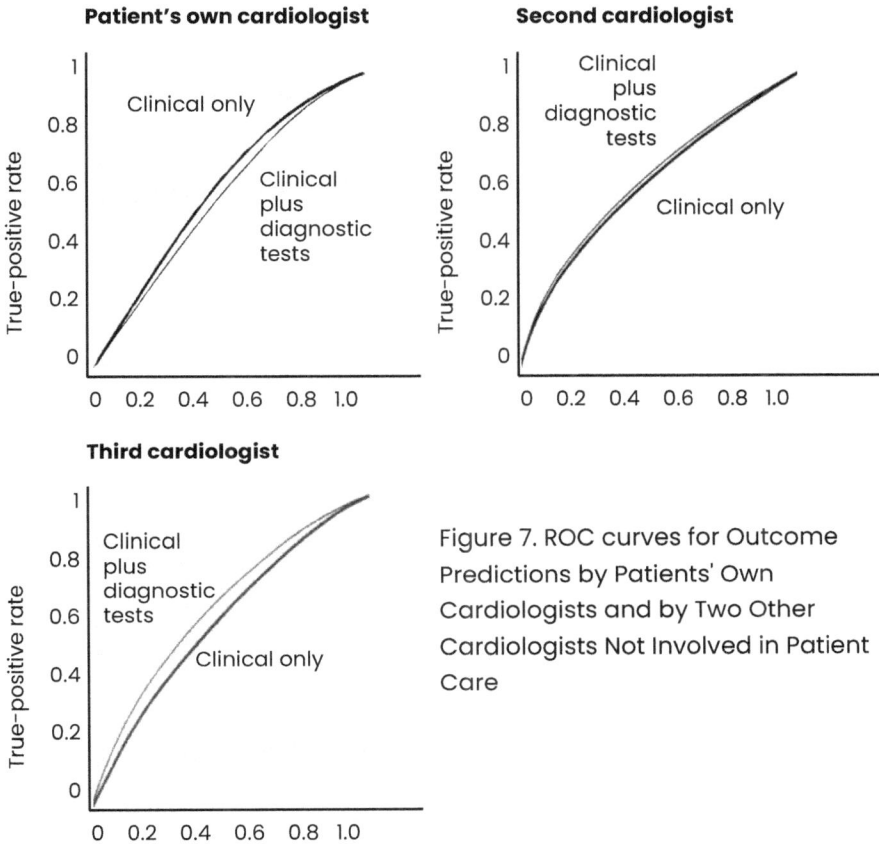

Figure 7. ROC curves for Outcome Predictions by Patients' Own Cardiologists and by Two Other Cardiologists Not Involved in Patient Care

At follow-up one year later, 24 patients had died from a cardiovascular cause and three others had suffered another heart attack. The predictions with and without the additional tests were virtually identical (see figure), being about 63 percent accurate, which was still a little better than chance (50 percent). We therefore concluded that the cardiologists only needed the basic clinical information to identify the higher risk patients. The more expensive and potentially harmful extra investigations were of no added benefit to either the physicians or the patients.

This study was published in *The Lancet* (45), a widely read British medical journal. I cannot prove that these results were responsible for a reduction in the number of unnecessary tests performed on heart attack patients in clinical practice. However, within a few years, these particular tests were no longer part of the routine care of heart attack patients in Canada.

As a caution, I should add that the use of coronary angiography in patients with heart attacks or angina is different from the routine use of the tests cited above. Coronary angiography can be quite helpful in determining if more specific interventions should be performed in order to improve the outcome of patients. For this reason, this investigation is now frequently performed in the majority of patients admitted with prolonged angina (chest) pain or a heart attack.

TWENTY

Exercise Training in Patients with Heart Failure

I can't take credit for coming up with the idea for this next study. Even though I treated many patients with heart failure, I never developed much of a research interest in this condition. A colleague of mine at Sunnybrook had set up a Heart Failure Clinic, which made it possible for him to participate in some multicenter trials involving new treatments. However, he did not engage in any independent research. On several occasions, he raised the possibility that patients with heart failure might derive benefit from exercise training. At this time, the prevailing belief was that these patients should remain mostly sedentary and avoid excessive exertion. Otherwise, unnecessary physical activity might lead to more severe heart failure or other serious complications.

Not wanting to miss out on an opportunity to investigate a belief which was mostly unsupported by research, I decided to design a study for my colleague, who would then provide the patients and supervise their involvement in it. The design was somewhat unconventional, although not by any means unique. The usual approach would be to randomly assign patients to either an exercise program or to usual daily activities and follow everyone for recurrent heart failure and other outcome measures. However, we wanted to monitor the status of participants for up to 12 months and it would be unfair to maintain a control group for that length of time. Most patients participating in an exercise training study would want to do the actual training at some point and not just be in a control group. So, patients with moderately severe heart failure were randomized to the intervention, a formal exercise program, or to a control group, who were given a pseudo-exercise program involving low levels of exertion. The patients randomized to the exercise program continued with it for 52 weeks. After 12 weeks in the pseudo-exercise program, the control group entered the same program as the intervention group, also for 52 weeks. The primary end-points were several measures of exercise capacity and quality of life at 12 weeks. The combined results of the exercise program at 12 weeks for the intervention group were compared to the results of the initial 12 weeks of the low level, pseudo-exercise program of the control group. Using this study design, we were able to have a control group while still maximizing the number of subjects having the intervention, since all of the patients participated in the exercise program, with the control group starting it after 12 weeks of being relatively sedentary.

I was soon to learn a new lesson about conducting clinical research. My colleague had given me the idea for the study and he was to provide the subjects and supervise their involvement. He did not express much interest in writing the grant proposal to support the project, since this was more my area of expertise. After I while, I got the impression that he saw the study as being more mine than his. Coincidentally, he was becoming more involved in a multi-centre trial involving a new drug for the treatment of heart failure of the same severity as being evaluated in the exercise study. He gradually became more interested in his own new project and the number of patients referred for the exercise study began to decline. I don't recall exactly how many patients we had hoped to enroll, but it was certainly more than the 21 who ended up being recruited.

I suppose I had been somewhat naïve in expecting someone who was primarily an excellent clinical cardiologist and not a researcher to sustain an interest in what was becoming somebody else's study. I should add that the exercise training program was being conducted at the Cardiac Rehabilitation Centre outside of the hospital and neither of us actually participated in the exercise training or assessments of cardiorespiratory function. These tasks were performed by the staff in the Cardiac Rehabilitation Centre.

Despite the limited sample size of our study population, the project otherwise progressed as expected. My colleague did follow the patients from a clinical care perspective and I supervised the overall conduct of the study, ensuring that the appropriate protocols were being followed. All of the patients randomized either to starting with the exercise program or to first being control subjects completed the initial 12 weeks. Fifteen of the 21 patients successfully completed all 52 weeks of the extended study.

Reasons for withdrawal included worsening heart failure (three patients), non-fatal cardiac arrest (one patient) and other, non-cardiac conditions (two patients). The remaining 15 patients exhibited significant improvements in in their functional status and were considered to have benefited from the aerobic exercise training program. The improvements in cardiovascular function over 52 weeks (see Figure 8) included significant improvements in performance including peak oxygen intake, reduction in resting heart rate, ventilatory threshold (for the onset on anerobic metabolism) and peak power output on the stationary cycle.

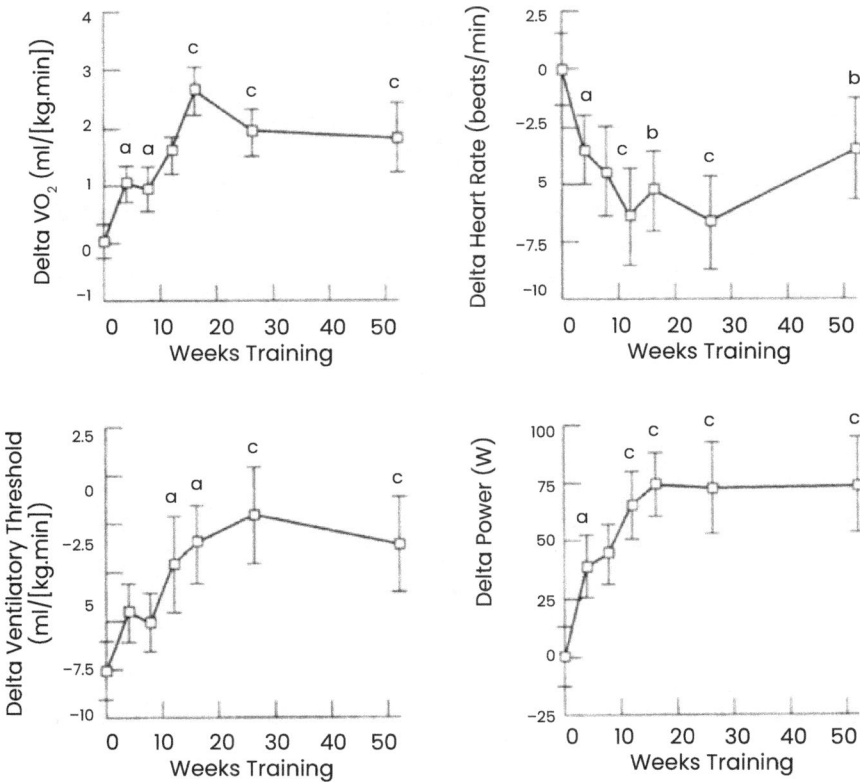

Figure 8. Improvements in Cardiovascular Fitness over 52 Weeks During Exercise Program.

I now started to prepare a manuscript for publication. By the time we had completed our study, including the 12 months of follow-up, at least one other article (46) on exercise training in 11 patients with heart failure had been published. Although this study had several methodologic concerns, it did appear to be a placebo-controlled experiment. Possibly because we were no longer the first to perform exercise training in this type of patient and because our study's design was somewhat unconventional, we had great difficulty getting the manuscript accepted for publication. Reviewers also seemed biased against the idea that these patients might benefit from exercise training. Furthermore, I was the senior author on the paper, which was appropriate considering my involvement in the study. However, I would not have been recognized by the experts in heart failure who reviewed the manuscript as being one of them. I would be the first to admit that all of the above is quite speculative. For whatever reason, I was left with a manuscript which had been rejected by four or five journals, something I was unaccustomed to seeing.

By now, I was quite discouraged and was prepared to forget about seeing these results published. Also, my cardiology colleague had left Sunnybrook for a non-teaching hospital in another city. However, the head of the Cardiac Rehabilitation Centre, Dr. Terry Kavanagh, had done a lot of work in supervising the aerobic training program of the participants. He was also a highly respected leader and researcher in cardiac rehabilitation. I decided to hand the manuscript over to him and moved on to my other research projects. To his credit, he extensively revised the paper, making the focus more on the physiologic aspects of the study and less on exercise training as a possible therapy for heart failure patients. He submitted the manuscript to the leading cardiovascular journal in his previous homeland, *Heart* (formerly the *British Heart Journal*), and it was accepted (46). I learned several lessons from this experience, the most important being that it was now time for me to concentrate on my research in hypertension.

Although this study was my only venture into heart failure, the rationale for subjecting patients with this condition to an exercise program was consistent with my other studies. In this instance, the reluctance to have these patients become more active was based more on theory than on research data. Once again, anyone could have recognized the need for a proper study. When my colleague first discussed his ideas with me, I immediately recognized another opportunity to answer an important question—was exercise good or bad for patients with severe heart failure? Based upon our own results and those of other similar studies, the answer is now an unequivocal "Yes, exercise is good."

TWENTY-ONE

Reporting Bias

In the 1990s, many patients receiving treatment for hypertension began to record their blood pressure at home using inexpensive devices purchased from a local pharmacy. The usual practice was for patients to write down readings recorded between office visits which were then shown to their doctor. Often these readings became the basis for adjustments to the patients' drug regimen. I suspected that most family physicians believed that these readings were the same as those which the device had actually recorded. However, being curious, I wondered if some, or perhaps all of the readings might be fictitious?

This question was definitely in my mind when the next generation of home blood pressure recorders became available. These new devices were capable of storing anywhere from 30 to 100 or more readings, which could then be downloaded by the patient or physician. Once again, I saw an opportunity for a study, this time to determine how many patients performing home blood pressure recordings were being truthful in documenting the readings they reported.

The study was easy to design. I only needed to have my assistant instruct patients having a 24-hour ambulatory blood pressure recording on the use of a home blood pressure recorder, which we provided. Following their initial ambulatory recording, the patients were given a form to keep track of their home blood pressure readings, which were to be taken in duplicate, twice daily for seven days. As you may have guessed, we did not tell the patients that the home recorder itself had a memory for storing the readings. We were careful to emphasize that the patient should not use the device to record any extra readings on themselves or on others.

However, there was a problem with this simple study which I had not considered and that is deception. When we submitted the proposal to the hospital's Ethics Review Board, the initial response was that we could not deceive the patients. However, I believed that if the patients knew the readings were being stored, they would be more likely to record the actual measurements. The protocol was sent out to several other ethicists for their opinions. The result was mixed, with no clear-cut answer as to what should be done. As a consequence, the Sunnybrook Ethics Review Board allowed us to proceed with the study without divulging the storage of readings to the patients.

A consecutive series of 39 patients who were also undergoing 24-hour ambulatory blood pressure monitoring were enrolled into the study. The average office blood pressure recorded by the patients' physicians was 159/91 mmHg compared to an average awake ambulatory reading of 149/89 and average home reading of 152/89 mmHg. The reported systolic and diastolic readings were compared to the readings actually recorded (see figure). Only seven of the patients reported readings which exactly matched those stored in the device. The average systolic blood pressure reported by nine of the patients was at least 10 mmHg different from the average value for the stored readings. Similarly, 14 patients had differences of at least 5 mmHg for the diastolic blood pressure. There was no clear pattern to the differences, with the reported readings sometimes being higher and sometimes lower. For this reason, the overall averages of the home and awake ambulatory blood pressures were similar. Readings that were reported as higher or lower than the actual readings tended to offset each other. For the individual patients, a difference of at least 10/5 mmHg was considered to be clinically important, such that it could affect making a diagnosis of hypertension or lead to an adjustment in the treatment regimen, if the patient was already taking therapy.

Part of our agreement with the Ethics Review Board was that we would not discuss any discrepancies in the two sets of readings with the patients. We were left to speculate on why some patients reported higher readings than actually taken and why others reported lower readings. One theory was that the individuals reporting the higher values were more concerned about their high blood pressure and wanted to convince the doctor that they should be treated. As for the lower readings, the patients may have been more concerned about possible side effects and reported lower readings in order to avoid having to take medication.

The results of our study were published in October 1998 (48). The following month, an almost identical study (49) appeared in a different medical journal with exactly the same findings. Dr. Thomas Mengden and colleagues had also used deception in order to demonstrate what we had called "reporting bias." Despite these two publications, the various guidelines for the use of home blood pressure measurements continued to ignore the possibility that the readings reported by patients might not be accurate.

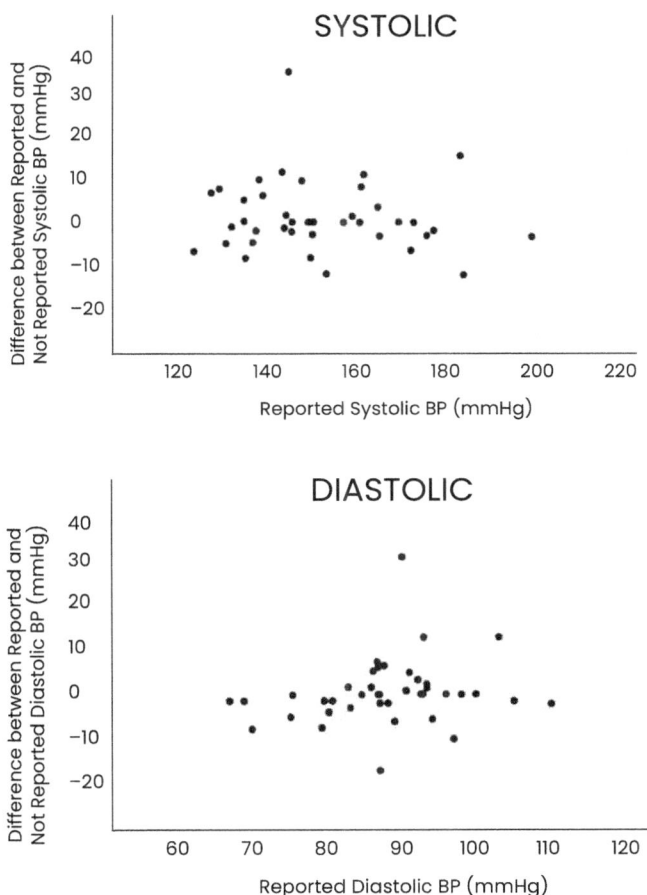

Figure 9. The difference between home systolic and diastolic blood pressure (BP readings reported correctly and readings taken but not reported, plotted against the reported values for each patient.

By 2014, I decided to try and rectify this ongoing problem. Together with a colleague, Dr. George Stergiou, we reviewed the studies which had subsequently examined various aspects of reporting bias (50). We found another seven articles on reporting bias which had been published since 1998. Patients in these studies were informed to a greater or lesser extent about the purpose of the study and the storage of readings to be compared to their reported values. None of the studies included the same level of deception that Dr. Mengden and I had used. Although the results were quite heterogeneous, there seemed to be a pattern. The more the patients knew about the storage of the blood pressure measurements, the more accurate were their own written readings.

Even now, the website of Hypertension Canada still includes a form for patients to use for writing down their home blood pressure readings which can then be shown to their family doctor. If you happen to be recording your blood pressure at home and want to have the maximum impact for your efforts, I would suggest that you bring your device to show the doctor the actual readings. Physicians are accustomed to relying on their own measurements, but showing them the actual home blood pressure readings is one way of increasing their value in the management of your hypertension.

TWENTY-TWO

24-hour Ambulatory Blood Pressure Monitoring

In April 1985, I became aware of a new device for recording blood pressure in patients carrying out their usual activities over the course of 24 hours. At this time, the diagnosis of hypertension was being made in the doctor's office using a stethoscope and a mercury sphygmomanometer (a column of mercury with markings on it from 0 to 300 mmHg). This technique had been in use since 1905, with virtually no changes, other than periodic guidelines on the proper method for obtaining readings. For example, in 1939, the American Heart Association published its first of a series of recommendations (51) which included having the patient rest before recording the blood pressure, using a properly calibrated instrument and being aware of irregular heart rhythm. By 1985, several publications were reporting that the blood pressure during usual daily activities might be lower than readings recorded manually in the office setting. This relationship did not make too much sense to me since one would expect blood pressure to be higher when the patient is more active and lower when resting quietly in a doctor's examining room.

The monitor for recording blood pressure over 24 hours used a new technique which involved transforming oscillations in the wall of the artery in the arm when the cuff was deflated into an electrical waveform. Each heartbeat created its own waveform which was then converted into a blood pressure reading using a special analytic technique. Preliminary studies had reported that this new method produced accurate readings which were similar to those obtained using the mercury sphygmomanometer under standardized conditions.

On a day when I had an appointment to see my dentist, I had my research assistant place the cuff on my upper arm and the attached 24-hour blood pressure monitor was hooked over my shoulder using a strap. One drawback was obvious. The recorder weighed several pounds, mainly because it used eight "C" batteries. I set the device to record my blood pressure every 15 minutes and wore it for 24 hours. When it came time to analyze the recording, I was surprised to see that my blood pressure had remained normal during my visit to the dentist and that the readings seemed quite accurate, with no obvious errors. Both the average daytime ambulatory reading and my blood pressure in the office were very normal. After further testing, I decided to purchase several of these 24-hour blood pressure recorders. In doing so, I became the first person to use ambulatory blood pressure monitoring in Canada.

From here onward, patients referred to my office by their family doctors for evaluation of possible hypertension began to have their readings recorded routinely over 24 hours in order to supplement the measurements obtained with the mercury sphygmomanometer.

There were two reasons why I did not embark on a research program using this new technology. First, I was already involved in a number of other studies, some of which I have already described. Second, I had recruited a colleague who also had an interest in hypertension and needed a project for his research. I introduced him to the 24-hour blood pressure recorder and he developed a research study to compare the readings to measurements taken in the office and after exercise. He was able to obtain funding for his study and started recruiting subjects. However, after collecting data on several hundred patients, he seemed to lose interest in academic medicine. After a promising start to his career, he left Sunnybrook for a position in the pharmaceutical industry.

Even though I had given over this area of research to my colleague, I had continued to use 24-hour blood pressure monitoring for my office patients. After a while, the differences I noted between the office readings and the measurements recorded over 24 hours became too interesting to ignore. Until then, virtually all of the research using 24-hour ambulatory blood pressure had involved using this new technology to make a more accurate diagnosis of hypertension before drug therapy was started. Instead of joining the others who were interested in white coat hypertension (high office blood pressure with normal readings on ambulatory blood pressure monitoring during usual daytime activities) in untreated patients, I decided to look at a different population, patients who were already receiving drug therapy for hypertension, with the diagnosis usually having been made by their family doctor on the basis of the office blood pressure. I was curious to know what might have

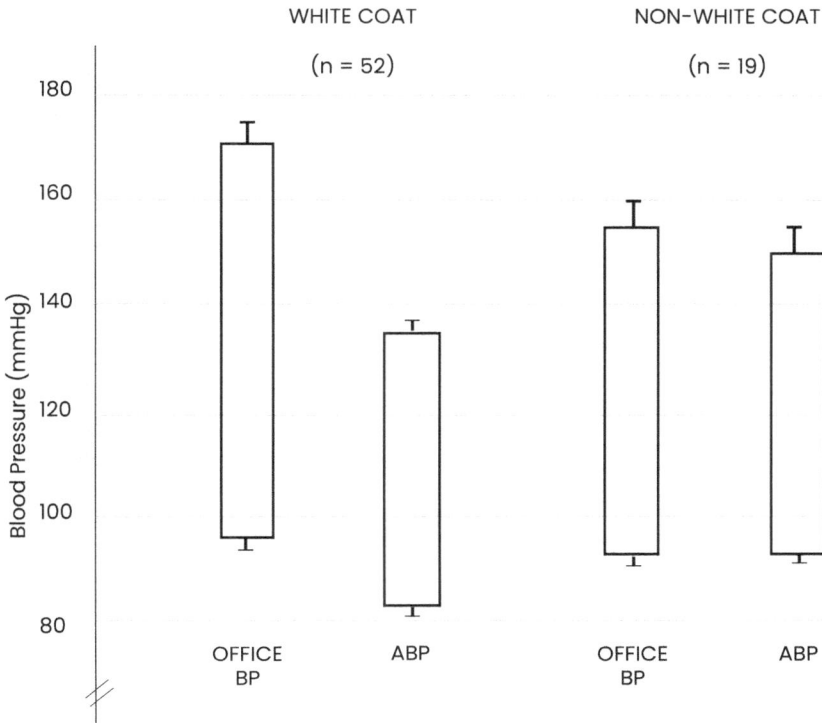

Figure 10. Mean office and ambulatory daytime blood pressure values for patients with and without white coat phenomenon.

happened to those individuals who had been treated for what might only have been white coat hypertension.

By 1990, I had data on 71 treated hypertensive patients, including the blood pressure recorded in my office and readings obtained using the 24-hour monitor during usual activities over a full day. Analysis of the data showed that 52 of 71 patients exhibited a white coat effect, which I defined as an average blood pressure at least 20/10 mmHg higher in the office compared to the awake ambulatory reading. The overall average reading recorded in the office (170/96) was considerably higher than the ambulatory blood pressure while awake (135/83).

Since actual blood pressure readings have not been mentioned for a while, I will explain again what the numbers mean. The first, higher number—systolic—represents the highest pressure inside the artery in the arm following a heartbeat. The second, lower number—diastolic—is the lowest pressure in the cycle prior to the next heartbeat. When readings are recorded with a stethoscope and a mercury sphygmomanometer, the higher number is detected by the appearance of sounds in the artery heard with the stethoscope and the lower number is recorded when the sounds disappear. As mentioned earlier, electronic devices, such as the one used to record readings over 24 hours, measure blood pressure from electronic signals and waveforms which develop as the cuff is deflated. Of interest, the white coat effect was associated with a disproportionate increase in the systolic blood pressure, which was consistent with our understanding that stress or exercise selectively increases the systolic reading more than the diastolic.

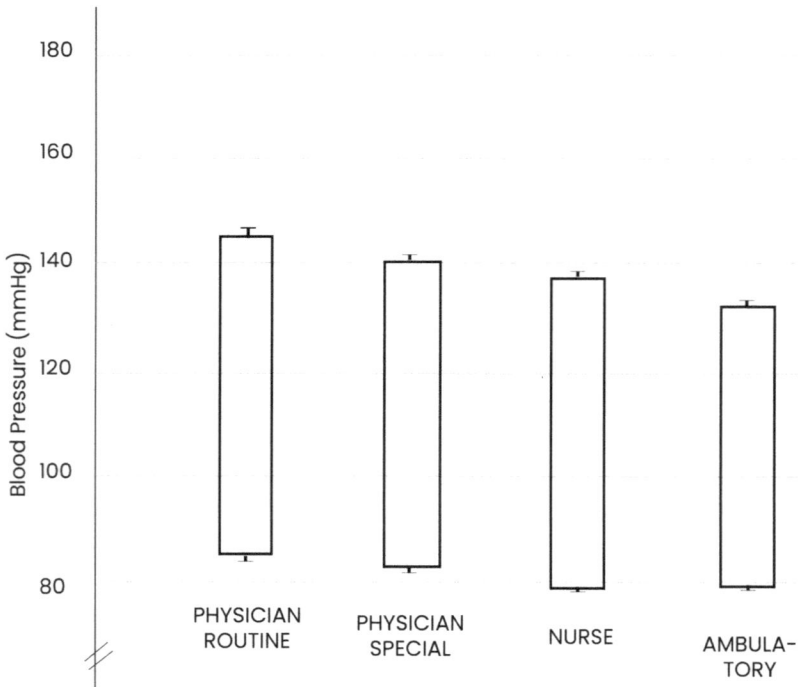

Figure 11. Mean (+/− SEM) blood pressure values are shown for measurements taken by the patients' own physician (special for the study and routine office readings), by the research nurse, and mean awake ambulatory blood pressure. All office readings with the exception of the nurse diastolic blood pressure were significantly different (P < .001) from the ambulatory blood pressure.

The initial series of 71 treated patients (52) undergoing 24-hour ambulatory blood pressure monitoring had been obtained from my own office practice. I wondered why there had been such a marked white coat effect, considering that my office nurse was recording the manual blood pressure properly, especially without conversing with the patient. It was also possible that family doctors had been selectively referring to me patients with apparent resistance to hypertension, due to having an underlying white coat effect. The next step would be to examine office readings in routine clinical practice.

As part of the study (53), my research nurse visited the offices of six family doctors in the community near our hospital. She examined the office charts and found a random sample of 147 patients who were being treated for hypertension. At their next visit, she obtained their informed consent to participate in the study. The protocol involved the documentation of several blood pressure measurements: the average of the office readings recorded by the family doctors during the previous three months (routine office blood pressure), the average of two readings recorded by the research nurse during two study visits about two weeks apart, a special reading performed just for the study by the patient's own family doctor and the mean awake blood pressure obtained from a 24-hour ambulatory recording. An ultrasound test of the heart (echocardiogram) was also performed on each patient in order to obtain a measure of the size of the pumping chamber (left ventricle) of the heart, which is often enlarged when high blood pressure is present.

In these treated patients, the family doctors' routine readings averaged 146/87 mmHg compared to a mean awake ambulatory blood pressure of 132/78 mmHg (see figure). It was also of interest that this patient population had a much lower mean routine office blood pressure (146/87) than the initial reading of 170/96 mmHg recorded by my nurse in our series of 71 patients. This finding tended to confirm my suspicion that the patients referred to my office had more severe hypertension which was resistant to drug therapy. (See Figure 12, next page.)

Further analysis of the data showed that the routine office blood pressure measurements in 91 of the 147 patients exhibited a white coat effect, with the systolic reading at least 20 and/or 10 mmHg higher than the average ambulatory blood pressure recorded during awake hours. However, the family doctor's special office reading taken only for study purposes exhibited a white coat effect in only 51 of 147 patients, compared to 91 of 147 patients during routine office visits. It was evident that the family doctors were capable of

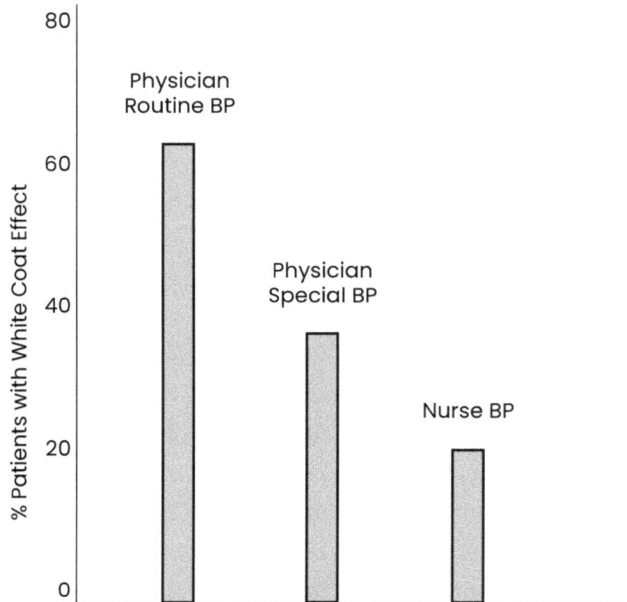

Figure 12. Percent of patients exhibiting a white coat effect based upon blood pressure (BP) measurements taken by the physician for the study (special), physician's routine office reading, and research nurse's reading.

recording an accurate blood pressure (BP for short), but were less likely to do so during routine office visits. Of interest, all of the readings were significantly correlated with size of the left ventricle (a measure of the effect of high blood pressure on the heart muscle), except for the doctor's routine office reading.

As my first decade of using ambulatory blood pressure monitoring in my practice was coming to a close, I began to think that white coat effect was more common in women. I decided to examine the prevalence of white coat effect by sex (54) in the 71 patients discussed above combined with another 81 referrals for ambulatory blood pressure monitoring. The overall mean manual office BP in this sample of 152 patients was 168/94 mmHg, compared to a mean awake ambulatory blood pressure of 141/85 mmHg.

A white coat effect (office blood pressure 20 and/or 10 mmHg higher than the awake ambulatory blood pressure) was present in 106 of the 152 patients. There was a white coat effect in 70 of 87 women in the study compared to only 36 of 65 men.

For this study, I defined a severe white coat effect as a difference of 40 and/or 20 mmHg, which was present in 49 of the patients. The sex differences were even more striking (see Figure 13), with severe white coat effect being present in 41 of the 87 female patients compared with only 8 of 65 men. Based upon these findings, we concluded that a white coat effect was more common in women, especially in an older age group. Subsequent studies reported over the next 25 years have been consistent with these observations.

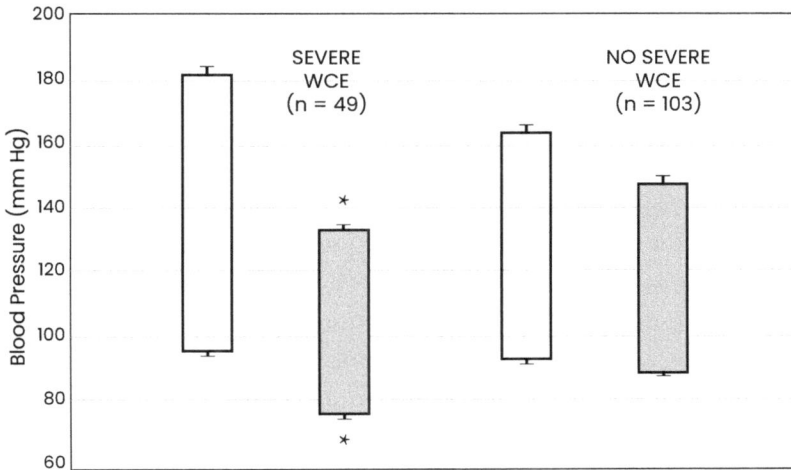

Figure 13. Mean office (white bars) and ambulatory (shaded bars) blood pressure values (+/− SEM) are shown for patients with and without a severe white coat effect (WCE). The asterisk (*) indicates P < 0.001 office vs. ambulatory blood pressure.

By 1998, I had come to the conclusion that there was now sufficient evidence to support a series of recommendations for the use of ambulatory blood pressure monitoring in clinical practice. Under the auspices of the Canadian Hypertension Society, I organized a meeting of specialists interested in blood pressure measurement, especially ambulatory blood pressure monitoring. After a thorough review of the scientific literature, we prepared a series of recommendations (55):

•   Physicians should only use ambulatory monitoring recorders which have been validated for accuracy independent of the manufacturer.

•   A decision to withhold drug therapy should take into account normal values for 24-hour and awake ambulatory blood pressure.

•   Ambulatory blood pressure measurements should be performed in untreated patients whenever white coat hypertension is suspected.

- Ambulatory blood pressure measurements should be performed in treated patients suspected of having a white coat effect.

- Changes in blood pressure recorded during sleep should be considered in making decisions regarding therapy.

These evidence-based recommendations were the first attempt to provide physicians with guidance on the use of ambulatory blood pressure monitoring. Perhaps because of a strict adherence to the evidence, these recommendations remain consistent with subsequent versions proposed by other national and international organizations.

Ambulatory blood pressure monitoring is now recognized as the best method for diagnosing hypertension. This recommendation is based upon the results of large studies which have shown that 24-hour blood pressure is significantly better than office readings in predicting future stroke and cardiovascular events. Until recently, ambulatory readings recorded during the daytime were the gold standard for determining an individual's blood pressure status. However, there has been a recent trend to relying more on the mean 24-hour reading, since the blood pressure during sleep is now considered to be the best predictor of future events.

TWENTY–THREE

Automated Office Blood Pressure Measurement

My studies on blood pressure measurement in the office and during 24-hour ambulatory monitoring had convinced me that we had a serious problem with how hypertension was being diagnosed in routine clinical practice. I had suspected that the high office readings in this setting were often due to the presence of the nurse or doctor who was taking the readings and usually also talking with the patient. Having now identified the problem and quantified its extent, I thought about how it might be corrected. An opportunity to study this white coat effect appeared when two family practice residents at our hospital needed to perform a research study as part of their training program. The design of the experiment was quite simple. We recruited 27 patients from the offices of nine doctors working in the hospital's Family Practice Unit. Each patient took two readings on their own using a home blood pressure recorder without anyone else being in the examining room. The patient's own family doctor also recorded two readings using a stethoscope and mercury sphygmomanometer. These readings could not be considered to be routine since the doctors were aware of their participation in a research study.

The results (see Figure 14 on the next page) were somewhat disappointing (56). The average blood pressure measurements recorded by the patients while alone using the patient-activated electronic recorder (157/83) were similar to the doctors' readings (155/80), with both being significantly higher than the average awake ambulatory blood pressure (145/78).

There were several possible explanations for why the patients' average reading was still higher than the awake ambulatory BP, the most likely being that the patients had to activate the electronic home blood pressure monitors at specific times by themselves, which might have created some anxiety. I was beginning to believe that the most accurate readings involved the least

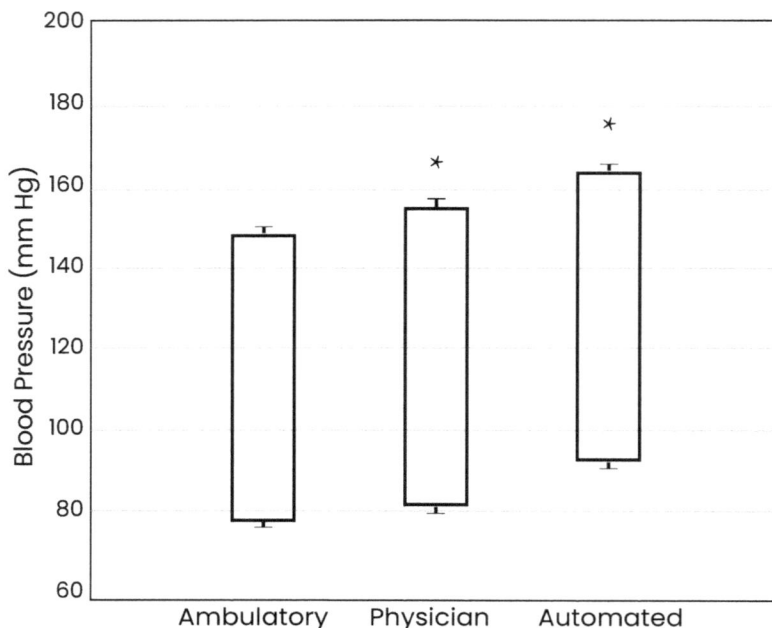

Figure 14. Mean (+/− SEM) systolic and diastolic BPs are shown for the physician, automated, and ambulatory recordings. The asterisk denotes a significant difference of P <0.05 between the ambulatory vs. physician or automated systolic BP.

human involvement, which was probably why the 24-hour ambulatory blood pressure was the best predictor of heart attack and stroke.

As in life, good fortune in research sometimes seems to fall from the sky, just as the apple landed on the head of Sir Isaac Newton. No doubt many others have suffered sore heads from falling apples, but Sir Isaac's head was like fertile soil, in that he was able to connect the falling apple to a new concept called "gravity."

Although I don't pretend to be Sir Isaac, a similar experience started me on a journey of 15 years which is now changing how doctors in the world record blood pressure in their offices.

After the failure of the experiment with self-measurement of blood pressure in the office, I had put aside the idea of eliminating human involvement from the process of recording office blood pressure. However, I had not forgotten what might be possible. Everything changed one day in 2002 when a family physician, Mark Gelfer, appeared in my office. While working in clinical practice in Vancouver, he had joined with a small Canadian technology company, VSM MedTech, to create an automated blood pressure recorder called the BpTRU. This device was similar to the usual home recorder, except that it was programmed to take five readings at one- or two-minute intervals after an initial test reading. The BpTRU was fully automated, with the five readings being recorded starting one minute after the activation button was pressed.

When I saw this device, I immediately thought of the earlier experiment with blood pressure self-measurement in the office. By using the BpTRU, it would now be possible to obtain five readings automatically without any involvement of the patient, who could be resting alone in a quiet room. Soon after being introduced to the BpTRU, I began to use it on new patients referred with hypertension to see if their readings would be different from what my assistant was obtaining using a mercury sphygmomanometer. All the patients also had a 24-hour ambulatory blood pressure recording as part of the usual routine for diagnosing hypertension in my office.

A total of 22 patients were enrolled in this preliminary evaluation of the BpTRU (see Figure 15). The average reading recorded by me was 174/92 mmHg compared to 155/88 mmHg for readings recorded with the BpTRU

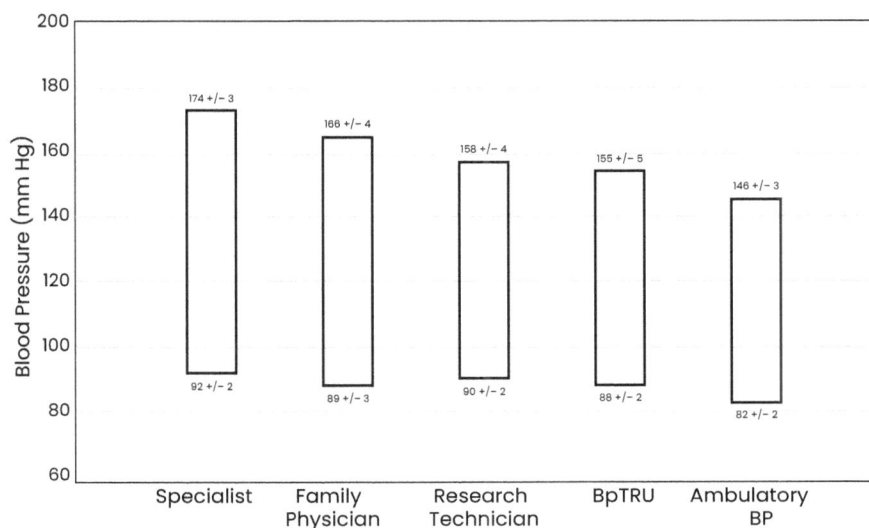

Figure 15. Mean (+/− SEM) blood pressure (BP) values obtained by the hypertension specialist, patient's family physician, research technician, and the automated BP recording device (BpTRU), along with awake ambulatory BP recordings.

while the patients were alone. (The systolic reading is the number most affected by any increased anxiety experienced by the patient.) The mean awake ambulatory blood pressure was 146/82 mmHg. Although the systolic reading recorded using the BpTRU was higher than normal (less than 140), it was still considerably lower than my own specialist's reading.

The BpTRU had eliminated most of the white coat effect seen with the manual reading. I reported these results at the annual meeting of Hypertension Canada in October 2002 and published the findings a few months later (57).

Shortly thereafter, Dr. Marshall Godwin, a family doctor doing research in hypertension at Queen's University in Kingston, Ontario, decided to investigate further the use of the BpTRU in hypertensive patients being treated by family physicians. From my presentation in 2002, he had become aware of the importance of leaving patients alone during the office readings. He sent a study nurse out to each family doctor's office to record a set of BpTRU readings and also to obtain a 24-hour ambulatory blood pressure recording from patients being treated for hypertension. In addition, the nurse was able to obtain the average of the patients' last three routine manual blood pressure readings recorded by their own family doctors. In 481 patients, both the average awake ambulatory systolic blood pressure and the systolic reading recorded using the BpTRU were about 10 mmHg lower than the average reading recorded during routine visits to the doctors' offices. Godwin's findings were reported in a somewhat obscure (at least for me) general medical journal (58), presumably read by family doctors, but not usually seen by hypertension specialists.

I don't recall who brought this article to my attention, but when I saw it soon after its publication in 2005, I experienced my second "apple-on-the-head" moment. For two years I had been dabbling with the BpTRU, using it record the office blood pressure in my own patients, while being involved in several other research studies. Upon reading Godwin's article, I immediately saw the possibilities for using the BpTRU in everyday clinical practice. I had missed out on the early days of research using 24-hour ambulatory blood pressure monitoring. I would not make the same mistake twice by missing out on studying these fully automated office blood pressure readings further.

TWENTY-FOUR

The CAMBO Trial

Not too long after, I received a telephone call from Dr. Norman Campbell in Calgary, who told me that he was working with several family physicians, including Dr. Godwin, to see if they could collaborate on a national research study on hypertension. I was asked to join a telephone conference call which had already been arranged to provide an opportunity for the group to discuss possible ideas for a project.

By coincidence, my colleague, Dr. Frans Leenen, who was now doing hypertension research in Ottawa, called to tell me about a new opportunity for research funding being offered by the Heart and Stroke Foundation of Ontario. Each year, the Foundation accepted applications for the possible funding of research studies which were then evaluated by a committee of experts in heart disease and stroke. The committee's job was to rate the grant proposals and to recommend those of highest quality for funding. In 2005, the new president of the Foundation decided to create a separate grant competition in order to award several groups of researchers much larger amounts for studies of particular interest to the Foundation. Dr. Leenen had just been successful in receiving money to perform a survey of blood pressure readings using the BpTRU device in residents of Ontario who were living in the community (59).

The topic the Foundation had selected for the second grant competition was "systolic hypertension" (high systolic combined with normal diastolic blood pressure readings). Systolic hypertension is a common type of high blood pressure which is mostly experienced by older patients whose diastolic readings are often normal. I immediately thought of the BpTRU and how it had reduced the systolic readings in the preliminary study I had done in 2002. Godwin's study had also reduced the systolic blood pressure disproportionately more than its effect on diastolic pressure. Perhaps the topic for the research study could be "systolic hypertension in the elderly."

Within a few days, we had our telephone conference and I proposed that we perform a multi-centre study comparing the management of patients who were being treated for systolic hypertension using either measurements recorded with the BpTRU or conventional readings obtained in the usual way with a mercury sphygmomanometer. The link to the grant competition would be that we would focus on systolic blood pressure as our primary outcome.

Instead of randomizing patients to one of these two methods of blood pressure measurement, we would randomize the doctors to use only one of these methods for their study patients. In doing so, we would minimize any bias which could arise if the same doctor recorded the blood pressure of different study patients using the "old" mercury sphygmomanometer or the new BpTRU. None of the other participants in the telephone conference offered an alternative proposal. The idea of responding to the request for proposals with a prospective, randomized controlled clinical trial involving the BpTRU was received with great enthusiasm. We proceeded to submit a summary of the study to the Foundation which was one of eight proposals selected for the submission of a more detailed grant application.

Since the proposal had been my idea, the task of writing the grant proposal landed on my desk. The first problem was that my colleagues on the conference call were working in several provinces, but the money would be coming from the Heart Foundation in Ontario. Giving money raised by volunteers in Ontario to researchers in Alberta and Quebec would probably not be acceptable. The problem was partly solved when Dr. Campbell in Calgary opted out of the study because of too many other commitments. I was left with Dr. Godwin in Kingston and Dr. Martin Dawes who was the Head of Family Medicine at McGill University in Montreal as collaborators.

My recent experience working with family physicians in my own city of Toronto had not been very positive. The study in six family doctors' offices published in 1995 had gone well, but several of my subsequent projects involving local family doctors had encountered more difficulty in recruiting patients. I needed to look beyond the confines of my own city for potential subjects. A colleague came to my rescue by suggesting that I visit Dr. Janusz Kaczorowski, a researcher in the Department of Family Medicine at McMaster University in Hamilton. I recall traveling to Hamilton on a snowy day in March to find him in an office far from any hospital or campus, in what looked like an industrial compound. Once we started talking, the surroundings no longer mattered. Dr. Kaczorowski had an unusual background, having left Poland in 1980 where he had been attending university and ultimately ending up in Montreal, where he obtained a Ph.D. in Sociology. While in Montreal, he got involved in some studies involving patients, which gave him an opportunity to apply his training in research and statistics. With this background, he went on to become the Director of Research in the Department of Family Medicine at McMaster University. We met for over an hour, during which time I reviewed our plans for the study. He not only readily understood what we were doing, but also offered several useful suggestions. Without any hesitation, I asked if he was interested in collaborating with us in this project and he accepted the offer.

By this time, I had chosen the possible sites for the study. Dr. Godwin would recruit patients in the city of Belleville which was near Kingston, Dr. Dawes would do the same in Montreal and Dr. Kaczorowski would be responsible for supervising the doctors in Brantford, a city west of Hamilton. With only one site outside of Ontario, I thought we had a chance at receiving funding for the project.

I am not sure who at the Foundation evaluated the eight proposals to make a final decision on funding, but I do know that the Scientific Committee, which was usually responsible for evaluating proposals submitted to the Foundation's annual grant competition, was not involved. Despite having a site in Montreal, our proposal was successful and we were given $1.5 million and up to five years to complete the study. This was a huge amount for a single research grant in Canada. The process by which it had been awarded was quite upsetting for members of the Scientific Committee of the Foundation, who had not been consulted. Nonetheless, the decision had been made by the president of the foundation and it was final.

I was reasonably confident that we could complete the project successfully. My colleagues had each been principal investigators of major studies in the past and were quite keen on moving forward with this one. We had already accomplished our first two tasks, getting financial support and agreeing on a name for the study: The **C**onventional versus **A**utomated **M**easurement of **B**lood Pressure in the **O**ffice (CAMBO) trial. However, before we even recruited a single patient our plans were turned upside down.

Dr. Kaczorowski announced that he had accepted the position of Director of Research in Family Practice at the University of British Columbia and would shortly be moving to Vancouver. At this early stage, I had the option of telling him that he could no longer be involved in our project, since he would be unable to supervise the doctors in Brantford. However, I had been so impressed by Dr. Kaczorowski's knowledge of research that I decided to keep him as a co-investigator, anticipating that he would be useful in helping us deal with issues which would inevitably arise during the conduct of the study. In Dr. Kaczorowski's absence, Dr. Sheldon Tobe, a kidney specialist at my hospital with an interest in hypertension, would now assist in supervising the family doctors in Brantford.

The other surprise involved Dr. Godwin, who had been working in Kingston for 12 years. He also had decided to accept another position, as Director of Research in the Department of Family Medicine at Memorial University in St. John's, Newfoundland. Not only had I lost the supervisor of the doctors in Belleville, I was also faced with another collaborator working outside of Ontario. Dr. Tobe and I were now the only investigators remaining in the same province as the Heart and Stroke Foundation of Ontario.

The move to St. John's did have an upside. Dr. Godwin agreed to continue in the study and to create sites in St. John's and Corner Brook, another city in Newfoundland. To my relief, the Foundation also agreed to continue funding this now national project with one of the largest research grants they had ever awarded.

The next step was to hire research nurses whose task it would be to recruit family physicians into the study. Initially, I was concerned that finding family doctors interested in participating would be as difficult in the smaller cities as it had been in Toronto. From my past experience, I knew that the secret to success would be finding a way to bypass the secretary in order to speak directly to the doctor. In Toronto, this stage had been a major obstacle, since the secretaries were very protective of their doctors. So, in hiring research nurses, we intentionally selected individuals who had either previously worked for a local physician or who were currently working in a practice on a part-time basis. Using this approach, there was no longer any concern about gaining access to the doctors, since their secretaries and nurses considered the research staff to be "one of their own."

The recruitment pattern in each city was quickly established. Once the study nurse got the first physician's agreement to participate, his name was then used when introducing the study to the next practice. In calculating the minimum number of patients required for the study, we realized that recruitment would need to be gradual, over a period of two years. It was important to maintain a manageable workload for the study nurses, who needed to visit the doctors' offices frequently to collect data and to ensure the patients remained in the study. Patients were followed for two years, with the 24-hour ambulatory blood pressure recording being performed three times, at the beginning of the study and after the first and second year. Although the follow-up period was two years, we were most interested in the readings taken on the first visit after enrollment. At this time, the patients would still be taking their previous medications, so we would be able to compare blood pressure readings recorded during routine office visits before enrollment to readings obtained with the BpTRU during the first study visit. By now, office blood pressure recorded using devices such as the BpTRU were called "automated office blood pressure" (AOBP).

A total of 555 patients under the care of 88 physicians who worked in 67 practices were enrolled into the study. The results (60) confirmed our initial hypothesis. The use of the automated BpTRU recorder taking multiple readings with the patient resting alone in a quiet place eliminated the white coat effect. During the first office visit of the patients randomly allocated to having their blood pressure recorded using the BpTRU, the average reading was 14.3/4.0 mmHg lower than it had been during the last routine visit prior to enrollment in the study. The corresponding difference in the control, manual blood pressure group was 8.0/1.5 mmHg. The magnitude of the differences between the two groups was statistically significant.

The observed fall in blood pressure in the control group was a concern, but was not unexpected. Involvement in a research study often changes the behavior of the patient and/or the doctor. For this reason, we had randomized each doctor's practice to either an intervention group or a control group. Two separate consent forms were given to the doctors and to patients in the AOBP and control groups in order to minimize any changes in behaviour. Even though we did not tell the physicians and nurses in the control practices anything about the AOBP intervention, they still knew they were being watched, simply because they were now in a research study. Such observation often improves performance, but, in this instance, the readings were only lower, but were not more accurate. Lower because persistently high readings on drug therapy would tend to reflect poorly on their care and the doctors and nurses would prefer not to reveal this to others. The return visit after enrollment was an opportunity for the office staff to revise the readings downward. In most instances, this lower reading was likely made subconsciously.

We knew that the readings were probably not more accurate because 50 percent of the manual readings were still being rounded off to the nearest zero value, compared to only 14 percent in the AOBP group. Also, unlike the AOBP, the manual readings still correlated poorly with the awake ambulatory blood pressure. The difference between the AOBP and manual blood pressure groups persisted during the two years of follow-up (61), with the average readings in both groups gradually becoming somewhat lower because more medications were being prescribed to the patients in both groups.

The CAMBO trial was not a perfect study. By design, the investigators had to rely on the family physicians and their nurses to follow the protocol and record the AOBP properly. The study nurses only came by after the patients' visits and could not correct any problems which might have occurred beforehand. Very few randomized, controlled clinical trials have been performed successfully in routine clinical practice, perhaps because the staff collecting the data do not have the same commitment to the study as do the investigators. To be fair, the doctors and nurses in the community are usually quite busy seeing multiple patients with a variety of disorders and might sometimes find it difficult to devote the time required to follow a specific protocol.

Nonetheless, it was important to demonstrate that AOBP produced office readings which were more accurate and closer to the average blood pressure during usual daily activities, as recorded by the 24-hour ambulatory recorder. Evidence from randomized, controlled clinical trials is considered to be of utmost importance when it comes to evaluating the validity of new treatments, or, as in this case, new techniques for diagnosing a condition such as hypertension.

Other Studies Performed Concurrently with CAMBO

The $1.5 million grant provided by the Ontario Heart Foundation allowed us to perform a series of other experiments to evaluate various aspects of AOBP. Given my background in clinical pharmacology which involved the assessment of new drug treatments, I decided to approach the BpTRU device as one would a new drug. The CAMBO trial represented a typical stage in new drug development, one in which the treatment is compared to a placebo or usual therapy, if another drug is already being used to treat the condition of interest. In this instance, the mercury sphygmomanometer was the equivalent of "usual therapy" in that had been used for one hundred years to measure blood pressure.

In the first of these studies (62), I noted the change in blood pressure during each of the six readings recorded by the BpTRU to see how rapidly the decrease occurred. In new drug development, this protocol is the equivalent of an acute dosing study, in which the time-course of the effect, such as a fall in blood pressure with a new medicine for hypertension, is documented. An initial "test" reading is performed in the presence of the doctor or nurse and fulfills several purposes. It confirms that the cuff is in the proper position on the patient's arm and that the device is recording a valid blood pressure reading. It also gives the hypertension specialist some indication of the reading a family doctor might obtain during a routine office visit. Finally, the difference between this first reading and the second one with the patient resting alone in the quiet room gives an indication of how quickly the white coat effect can disappear after the patient is left alone.

In 50 patients, the average difference in blood pressure between the first test reading (162/85 mmHg) and the second "alone" reading was 15/4 mmHg. The next alone reading was 4/1 mmHg lower with the remaining three readings being only slightly lower. The average of the five alone readings was 142/80 mmHg. Thus, the white coat effect associated with the presence of office staff was mostly eliminated within one to two minutes of the patient being alone. Although this degree of white coat effect was expected, we did not anticipate it disappearing so quickly. It should be noted that the first reading with the patient alone was recorded after a one-minute delay, which allowed time for the nurse or doctor to leave the room.

For new drugs, it is also important to know the most appropriate interval between doses, which helps to determine how many times a day the medicine should be taken. When it came to the BpTRU, I was interested in knowing if readings taken at one-minute intervals would produce the same results as those recorded every two minutes. In the first experiment, 200 patients referred for 24-hour ambulatory blood pressure monitoring had the five readings taken at one-minute intervals. For the next 200 patients, we used the setting for two-minute intervals. For both intervals, the BpTRU device times the readings from the start of one reading to the start of the next one. All 400 patients also underwent 24-hour ambulatory blood pressure monitoring. The differences between the awake ambulatory blood pressure and office readings taken with the BpTRU every one minute and every two minutes were similar.

In another 50 patients, AOBP was recorded twice, before and after a 24-hour ambulatory blood pressure recording. Patients were randomized to have the readings recorded on the first day at either one- or two-minute intervals, with the opposite setting after the 24-hour ambulatory BP. The differences between the mean awake ambulatory blood pressure and the one- and two-minute AOBP were once again similar. On the basis of these findings, I concluded (63) that AOBP readings can be taken at one-minute intervals. We could now say that it took less time to perform AOBP readings than it would take to measure blood pressure the usual way with the mercury sphygmomanometer. However, this comparison was only valid if the manual reading recorded using the mercury device included at least five minutes of rest before the first reading. AOBP measurements did not require this additional period of rest.

In the next study (64), I wanted to evaluate the consistency of AOBP readings from one visit to another and also in different settings. Manual blood pressure is known to vary depending on the setting in which readings are taken. Since AOBP involved little or no human involvement, perhaps the setting for readings would be less important. In this study, 62 consecutive patients had AOBP performed in my office before and after referral for 24-hour ambulatory blood pressure monitoring. An AOBP was also performed by the ambulatory blood pressure monitoring technician prior to attaching the recording device. All three sets of AOBP readings were within 1 mmHg of the average systolic and diastolic values of the awake ambulatory blood pressure. Thus, AOBP is consistent from visit to visit and readings exhibit a close relationship to the awake ambulatory blood pressure, which is the gold standard for an accurate blood pressure measurement.

Around this time, my colleagues were publishing articles based on data obtained with 24-hour ambulatory blood pressure monitoring in hundreds of patients. When I expressed frustration at not having similar data for AOBP, a close colleague asked: "What about all the patients who come to your unit for 24-hour blood pressure monitoring? Haven't you also been doing AOBP routinely on them?" This suggestion led to several more studies.

My objective was to make this as much as possible a reflection of what might be happening in routine clinical practice. So, I first got permission from the hospital's Ethical Review Board to collect basic information on referrals for ambulatory blood pressure monitoring without a consent form, including the family doctor's last blood pressure reading prior to booking the appointment. Only my technician saw these patients, since the purpose of the visit was to do the 24-hour blood pressure recording and not to see a hypertension specialist.

The first publication (65) using this new database involved 309 patients who had an average blood pressure of 152/87 mmHg on the last routine visit to their family doctor. Their average AOBP was 132/75, which was similar to the awake ambulatory blood pressure of 134/77 mmHg. As in the CAMBO trial, the awake ambulatory blood pressure readings also correlated significantly better with the AOBP than did the routine manual office blood pressures reported by the family doctor. These results were striking, considering that the family doctor's blood pressure was the basis for starting treatment and for increasing medication, if the readings were high.

The following year, I performed a follow-up study (66) on another 300 patients who were also referred for 24-hour blood pressure monitoring. In this study I was interested in comparing the AOBP to readings obtained by the patient's own self-measured readings at home, using an automated home blood pressure recorder. The initial results were somewhat surprising in that the awake ambulatory blood pressure and self-measured blood pressure at home were similar. However, the average BpTRU reading was lower.

I sought an explanation for this finding by dividing the patients into those with a normal blood pressure and those with hypertension, some of whom were receiving treatment with medication. Patients were divided into normal and high blood pressure based upon manual readings which had also been recorded by my research technician. In the 139 patients with high manual BP readings, the mean AOBP, home blood pressure and awake ambulatory blood pressure were all similar. Conversely, in the subjects with a normal manual blood pressure, the AOBP was much lower than the other readings, which explained why the AOBP in the entire group of 300 patients had been relatively lower.

At the time, I did not pay much attention to the observation that the AOBP was lower than the awake ambulatory blood pressure and home blood pressure in normotensive patients. I would have to wait another 10 years before realizing that this finding was actually quite important (67). Meanwhile, the idea of using a less expensive home recorder to replace the BpTRU was set aside, since having a hypertensive patient being involved in the blood pressure measurement process seemed to cause the readings to be higher, as it had also done in our 1997 study (56). It was now evident that patient involvement in taking the blood pressure in itself could create a white coat effect.

By now, the CAMBO study was almost completed, so I undertook one final experiment using the remaining funds. Until now, the only devices for recording AOBP were the BpTRU and Omron 907, which I had previously evaluated. However, a third AOBP recorder was now gaining popularity in Europe, the WatchBP Office. This device recorded three blood pressure readings at one-minute intervals with the patient resting alone. There was a one-minute delay before the first reading which gave the office staff time to leave the room.

A 24-hour ambulatory blood pressure recording and AOBP reading recorded by the WatchBP Office device were obtained in 100 patients who had been referred to the ambulatory blood pressure monitoring unit. The average AOBP was 139/80 compared to an awake ambulatory blood pressure of 137/79 mmHg (68). Although the readings were quite similar, I did miss noticing what in retrospect might have been an important observation. If the first AOBP reading, which was a little higher, was discarded, the average of the second and third readings, 136/78, was even closer to the ambulatory blood pressure. This smaller difference is consistent with the approach taken by many physicians when recording office or home blood pressure, that is, to discard the first reading and use the average of the next two measurements as the patient's blood pressure.

By now, it was 2011. The CAMBO trial had been completed and the results published in the *British Medical Journal* (60), which guaranteed that the findings would be read by a large international audience of physicians. I had also been quite frugal with the funds provided by the Heart and Stroke Foundation of Ontario. Somehow, there was still money remaining from the initial $1.5 million grant and I was able to return almost $300,000 to the Foundation to be used by other researchers.

Following the publication of the results of CAMBO, I expected that the Canadian guidelines for measurement of blood pressure in the office would now recommend AOBP as the preferred method. We had clearly shown that blood pressure readings recorded during routine office visits were inaccurate and subject to a white coat effect, which would lead to an over-diagnosis of hypertension in 20 percent to 25 percent of patients. However, I underestimated the resistance to changing from manual blood pressure measurement, which had been in use for over a century. The only change in the 2011 Canadian guidelines (69) was a statement recognizing AOBP as an "alternative" to the conventional manual method for recording blood pressure. At the annual meeting of the guidelines committee, the criticism seemed directed more at me than at the data supporting the use of AOBP in clinical practice. By then, I had probably become too closely associated with AOBP. Canadians may treat success in medicine the same as they do with performing artists. In this respect, we are all no different than lobsters:

A couple waiting for their table in a restaurant in Manhattan noticed that there were two tanks of lobsters, but only one tank had a lid on it. The man asked the hostess why only one lid. She replied that the tank with a lid contained American lobsters. If not for the lid, they would climb out. The other tank had Canadian lobsters. As soon as one tried to climb out, the others would pull it back inside.

AOBP outside of Canada was criticized from a variety of perspectives. It took too long to take a reading (not true), doctors might not have a quiet place for the patient to be alone (existing guidelines already required such a place for five minutes of rest before manual blood pressure readings), the devices for recording AOBP were relatively expensive (true, but well worth the cost considering the benefits to patients) and there was a lack of data showing that AOBP was good for predicting the risk of future cardiovascular events.

This last criticism was true, but was also irrelevant, in that it involved AOBP being compared to 24-hour ambulatory blood pressure monitoring and, to a lesser extent, to home blood pressure. There was strong evidence that the ambulatory blood pressure was the best technique for estimating an individual's risk of experiencing a heart attack or stroke in relation to their blood pressure status. In 2011, there was also evidence supporting home blood pressure, but it was much weaker and still of somewhat uncertain value. The comparison of AOBP to these two methods of blood pressure measurement was irrelevant, in that the ambulatory and home techniques were being recommended for making a diagnosis of hypertension. According to the guidelines, office blood pressure should only be used for screening patients for possible hypertension, with the diagnosis to be confirmed by ambulatory or home blood pressure.

The real comparator for the use of AOBP in clinical practice should have been office blood pressure as it was being measured in routine clinical practice. The most appropriate study design would have involved the initial assessment of patients using both AOBP and a routine manual blood pressure reading, to be then followed for a number of years to determine if AOBP was a better predictor of future cardiovascular events. The problem with such a study is that as soon as a manual blood pressure was recorded as part of a research study, it would no longer have been routine. Readings obtained in a study are invariably taken with greater adherence to established guidelines for proper blood pressure measurement. There was already ample evidence, including from the control group in the CAMBO trial, that a manual blood pressure in a research study was not the same as one recorded in the "real world," with the latter being higher and usually less accurate.

TWENTY-SIX

The Cardiovascular Health Awareness Program

You will recall that I had decided to keep Dr. Janusz Kaczorowski involved in the CAMBO trial, even though he had moved to Vancouver before the first patient was enrolled. At the time, I had recognized that he might be useful in helping to analyze the data we would be collecting and in preparing a manuscript based upon our findings. Although these expectations were confirmed, I did not anticipate that our partnership would evolve into a decade of collaboration to advance the acceptance of AOBP in clinical practice.

Prior to leaving McMaster, Dr. Kaczorowski had been successful in receiving funding for the Cardiovascular Health Awareness Program (CHAP), which involved thousands of subjects in 39 medium-size communities in the province of Ontario (70). He randomized 20 of the communities to have residents over the age of 65 years undergo a cardiovascular assessment, which included an AOBP reading. Similar residents in 19 other communities did not have any special program and served as a control group. After 12 months, people residing in the communities in the intervention group had significantly fewer admissions to hospital for cardiovascular diagnoses than those living in the 19 control towns and cities. This reduction in cardiac events was attributed to better management of the subjects' blood pressure, which had been recorded more accurately using the AOBP technique.

When I discovered that the blood pressure in this program was being recorded using the BpTRU device, I saw an opportunity to perform a long-term follow-up to relate AOBP at the time of entry into the study to the risk of experiencing a future cardiovascular event. Dr. Kaczorowski accepted my proposal and continued to collect data on death and admissions to hospital from cardiac causes in over 10,000 subjects residing in the intervention communities. After almost five years of follow-up, we analyzed the outcome data, dividing the patients into two groups, those untreated for high blood pressure and those taking medications.

There were 3,627 community-dwelling residents aged over 65 years who were untreated for hypertension upon entry into CHAP (71). Residents in long-term care homes or in other institutions had been ineligible for the study. During an average follow-up of 4.9 years, 271 participants experienced a cardiovascular event, such as a stroke or heart attack. Analysis of the data showed that AOBP readings of 135/80 mmHg or greater were associated with a significantly higher risk of experiencing an adverse event. This threshold was consistent with the reading of 135/85 mmHg which had been used to define hypertension on the basis of the awake ambulatory and home blood pressure since our 1999 publication (54). Since systolic blood pressure is by far the most important determinant of cardiovascular risk, the small difference of 5 mmHg in the diastolic readings was considered to be of little importance. Thus, AOBP, awake ambulatory blood pressure and home blood pressure all had a similar threshold for defining hypertension on the basis of real cardiovascular events. In contrast, the comparable threshold for manual office blood pressure research studies was 140/90 mmHg, but in the community it was closer to 150/95 mmHg, since readings in routine clinical practice were subject to a white coat effect.

The remaining 6,183 participants in CHAP (72) had already been receiving drug therapy for hypertension when their cardiovascular status was evaluated, including an AOBP reading recorded using the BpTRU device. Our interest in these community residents on treatment for hypertension was to relate their AOBP reading to the likelihood of experiencing a cardiovascular event, in this instance over an average follow-up period of 4.6 years. As before, we focused on systolic blood pressure, which was the primary outcome of interest. In the final analysis, a systolic reading of 110–119 mmHg was associated with significantly lower cardiovascular events than either higher or lower AOBP readings. By then (2016), there was other evidence that the ideal blood pressure for most patients on treatment for hypertension should be a systolic reading of less than 120 mmHg. Our findings suggested that AOBP could be used to determine when the target office blood pressure for treating hypertension was reached.

On the basis of the findings from CHAP, CAMBO and the other AOBP studies, the 2016 Canadian hypertension guidelines (73) recommended AOBP as the "preferred" method for recording office blood pressure in clinical practice. AOBP was indicated for the screening of patients with possible hypertension, with the diagnosis to be confirmed with 24-hour ambulatory blood pressure monitoring, or, if not available, then with home blood pressure. AOBP could also be used to follow patients on drug treatment for hypertension so that appropriate changes in medication could be made.

TWENTY-SEVEN

AOBP Use by Family Physicians in Canada

Even before the 2016 guidelines were published, many family doctors in Canada had started to use AOBP to record office blood pressure in their patients. New diagnostic techniques are usually first used by specialists and then gradually move into clinical practice in the community. In the case of AOBP, the opposite occurred. Mark Gelfer, who had conceived the BpTRU, was a family doctor working in Vancouver. Marshall Godwin, who did the first major study with the BpTRU, was a family doctor affiliated with Queens University in Kingston, Ontario. Martin Dawes, who supervised the Montreal site in the CAMBO study, was Head of Family Medicine at McGill University and Janusz Kaczorowski was Director of Research in Family Practice at the University of British Columbia. Moreover, the CAMBO study involved 87 family doctors in five eastern Canadian cities. Early on, pharmaceutical companies had recognized that there was a demand for devices used to record AOBP, especially the BpTRU, which was relatively expensive. So, they frequently offered BpTRU recorders to family doctors who provided patients for research studies as compensation for their cooperation. We had done the same in the CAMBO trial. The only complaint we received was that we were unable to give each participating physician more than one recorder. Thus, it was not a coincidence that family doctors were the first to start using AOBP, before most specialists had realized its advantages.

When I gave lectures on AOBP, especially abroad, I was often asked how many doctors in Canada used AOBP. After a while, I saw an opportunity for another study, so I asked Dr. Kaczorowski if he could help me prepare a questionnaire to be sent to family physicians across Canada to learn more about how they record blood pressure in their patients. Even though Dr. Kaczorowski was not a medical doctor, all his research had been done with academic family physicians. By now, he had moved to Montreal where he was Director of Research in Family and Emergency Medicine at the University of Montreal. He was able to use his connections at the College of Family Physicians of Canada, the national regulatory body, to get access to the email addresses of family doctors across the country. We then designed a brief survey with several questions related to how blood pressure was being measured in the doctors' offices.

Although the results showed that family physicians did not always follow the Canadian guidelines for office blood pressure measurement, they were still quite positive. A total of 774 doctors selected at random from across Canada responded to the questionnaire. AOBP was used in 39 percent of patients who were being screened for possible hypertension. The good news was that hypertension was being diagnosed by manual blood pressure readings in only 21 percent of subjects, with 30 percent using AOBP, 22 percent home blood pressure and 14 percent ambulatory blood pressure. According to the Canadian guidelines, a diagnosis should have been done using either ambulatory or home blood pressure. It was somewhat disappointing to see only 14 percent of physicians using ambulatory recordings. Finally, 54 percent of doctors used AOBP to follow their patients after a diagnosis had been made. Thus, more than half of Canadian family doctors were using AOBP in their offices (74), and this was in 2016, before the guidelines recommending AOBP as the preferred method for office use had been published.

I am certain the percentage is currently much higher. I frequently ask people I meet how their doctor records their blood pressure and almost everyone says that an automated device is being used to take multiple readings while they are resting alone. This should not be surprising since about 13,000 BpTRU units were distributed in Canada, mostly to family doctors.

TWENTY-EIGHT

AOBP Outside of Canada

In 2017, AOBP got a major boost from the publication of a study (75) done in the United States, although later on this turned out to be a somewhat mixed blessing. The Systolic Blood Pressure Intervention Trial (SPRINT) was a multi-centre clinical trial involving 9,361 patients. It examined the benefits of treating hypertensive patients to achieve a target systolic blood pressure of either less than 140 mmHg or less than 120 mmHg. The results showed fewer cardiovascular events when treated to the lower target. From my viewpoint, the more interesting aspect of the study was that AOBP appeared to have been used to obtain office blood pressure readings. I say "appeared" because the procedure manual for the study clearly described the use of AOBP. However, a subsequent retrospective review (76) of how the research staff had actually recorded office blood pressure in the study suggested that only a quarter of the patients had a proper AOBP done, with various types of "almost" AOBP readings being taken in the other subjects. Regardless, it was evident that all of the office readings had been taken with greater care than in almost all other large clinical trials and that AOBP, or its equivalent, had been used in at least one-half of the patients.

A new set of American hypertension guidelines (77) appeared shortly after SPRINT was published. The lower target systolic blood pressure of <120 mmHg for treating most hypertensive patients was now recommended for clinical practice. Although the guidelines stated that AOBP was the best method for recording blood pressure in the office, it was not recommended as the preferred technique. Nonetheless, the fact that SPRINT had used a quasi-AOBP technique drew widespread international attention to AOBP, which by now was called "the Canadian method."

There was a specific reason why the 2018 American guidelines did not recommend AOBP. By the time the guidelines committee was close to completing its three years of review, another committee had been established by the American Heart Association with a mandate to update the previous AHA Statement on Blood Pressure Measurement, which had been published in 2005 (78). I was the only non-American member of the committee, presumably having been selected because of my work with AOBP. As expected, I was given responsibility for the section on office blood pressure. The committee had been instructed to base any new guidelines strictly on scientific evidence and not opinion.

Once on the committee, my objective was to have AOBP become the preferred method for blood pressure measurement in the U.S., as it already was in Canada. The evidence was clearly supportive of this position. My first task was to convince the committee chair, Dr. Paul Muntner, that this new technique for blood pressure measurement should replace the mercury sphygmomanometer. I provided him with copies of the articles on AOBP, including the CAMBO trial, and responded to numerous questions that he raised about the details of the various studies. My task was not always easy, in that Dr. Muntner was quite knowledgeable about clinical trials. He raised a number of issues, but all of them could be addressed with the available data. Finally, he agreed that AOBP had important advantages over current methods for performing office blood pressure.

The next step was to get the rest of the committee to agree. I can't say the decision to make AOBP the "preferred" method was unanimous, but a clear majority of the committee was supportive. The next step was to obtain approval at several levels at the American Heart Association. This process seemed to delay publication of the Statement on Blood Pressure Measurement for more than a year.

I later discovered that I was probably responsible for this delay. As part of my work on the committee, I had already collected all of the scientific articles on AOBP. I saw an opportunity to publish the results of this systematic review of the literature as a formal meta-analysis. (A meta-analysis involves combining data from a series of similar studies in order to increase the total number of subjects and, in this instance, their blood pressure readings, in order to provide more accurate findings.) Once again, my colleague, Dr. Kaczorowski, came to my assistance, by recommending Dr. Michael Roerecke to join us in doing the required complex statistical analyses. He was an unlikely co-author for an article on blood pressure, in that his appointment was at the Centre for Addiction and Mental Health in Toronto. Nonetheless, his skill in analyzing studies was applicable to any specialty. Dr. Roerecke proceeded to make a strong impression, by soon acquiring considerable knowledge about AOBP and the other types of blood pressure measurement.

By August 2018, we had completed our work, with the manuscript having been accepted for publication in the *Journal of the American Medical Association – Internal Medicine*. The publication of the meta-analysis supporting the use of AOBP would now be read by tens of thousands of family doctors and specialists in the United States. I was soon to discover why our AHA Statement on Blood Pressure Measurement had taken so long to be published. The American Heart Association had become aware of the meta-analysis, which would support their recommendation of AOBP as the preferred method for recording office blood pressure, and wanted to publish the Statement at the same time as the meta-analysis.

So, March 4, 2019 became a landmark day for both AOBP and me, in that both articles (79, 80) simultaneously appeared on this date. Moreover, I learned that there would also be an extensive promotion campaign by both the American Heart Association and American Medical Association to encourage American physicians to use AOBP. Interest in AOBP was further confirmed when I was invited to speak at the opening plenary session of the annual American Heart Association hypertension meeting in New Orleans. When I had finished speaking, one of the attendees took the microphone to say that he was working at one of the largest health maintenance organizations in the United States and that they were converting all of their blood pressure recorders over to AOBP. He added that 750,000 patients were already having their blood pressure recorded using AOBP and the number would soon be in the millions. Unlike in Canada, where use of AOBP had been spread via family doctors in the community, in the United States, use of the device would be incorporated into clinical practice mostly by several large health maintenance organizations, each having millions of members.

I was now considerably closer to achieving my objective of having AOBP become the preferred method for office blood pressure in the world.

However, the path toward this objective was never going to be smooth. The publication of SPRINT had catapulted AOBP into the forefront of a debate on how to measure office blood pressure. In a way, AOBP got caught in the crossfire. Many European experts in hypertension were highly critical of SPRINT. Their reasons were multiple and included the selection of AOBP for recording the patients' blood pressure and the lower target for treatment for the intervention group. Several influential members of the European hypertension community wrote editorials discouraging the use of AOBP. It was noteworthy that nobody questioned the evidence that AOBP was more accurate than blood pressure recorded in routine clinical practice, nor the fact that the average AOBP was identical to the average awake ambulatory blood pressure, a gold standard for determining the blood pressure status of patients.

The criticisms were mostly non-scientific. AOBP required a quiet place, such as an examining room, for the patient to sit. They claimed that most European offices did not have sufficient space for this and said that AOBP took 8–10 minutes (not true), which was said to be longer than a conventional office blood pressure. However, the European guidelines stipulated that conventional office blood pressure should include five minutes of antecedent rest in a quiet place (not needed with AOBP). The committee may have been acknowledging that most doctors do not currently let their patients rest for five minutes in a quiet place before recording their blood pressure, something which would explain why there was so much white coat effect in clinical practice. Another criticism was that the recording devices were too expensive, which was an indirect way of saying doctors didn't want to spend money in order to properly record blood pressure in their patients. Finally, they compared AOBP to 24-hour ambulatory blood pressure monitoring, which, as I previously noted, was inappropriate.

In 2018, the new European hypertension guidelines (81) suggested that AOBP might be the best method, but that it would not be recommended. This view was even a step backward from the 2013 European guidelines (82), which had stated that AOBP should be preferred, whenever feasible. Despite the obvious negativity in print, I was personally receiving very positive support from many of my European colleagues. Perhaps there was a fear of offending influential European experts who had not done research with AOBP and saw any improvements to office blood pressure as being a threat to their interests in 24-hour ambulatory or home blood pressure measurement. Another explanation might be that AOBP became a victim of a long-standing rivalry between American and European hypertension specialists.

TWENTY-NINE

Research Studies to Counter the Critics of AOBP

After the Canadian guidelines had recognized AOBP as the preferred method for recording BP in the office, I became convinced that it was only a matter of time before AOBP would achieve the same recognition in other countries' guidelines. The adoption of AOBP by the American Heart Association and American Medical Association confirmed my belief that the evidence favouring AOBP would eventually prevail, notwithstanding the disappointing recommendations from Europe. I decided to answer any publications portraying AOBP in a negative light with a combination of written commentaries and data from research studies.

My first effort actually pre-dated the 2016 Canadian guidelines, but was still quite useful in countering subsequent criticism of AOBP. Once again, I took advantage of an opportunity which had previously gone unnoticed. I remembered that Dr. Murray Matangi, a cardiologist in Kingston, Ontario, had been collecting data on AOBP and ambulatory blood pressure monitoring for many years. In a presentation at the European Society of Hypertension in 2009, he had reported that valid AOBP readings could be recorded in the office waiting room, provided that the patient was seated alone and left undisturbed while the readings were being taken. Dr. Matangi was primarily a clinical cardiologist and had not published his findings. When I pointed out that the data on AOBP in the waiting room deserved to be seen by a wider audience, he agreed to have me help him with further analysis leading to a publication (83).

Together, we examined AOBP data on 422 patients who had been referred to his office for 24-hour ambulatory blood pressure monitoring and a consultation for possible hypertension. The subjects included 248 treated hypertensive patients and 174 on no medication. We compared AOBP readings with the awake ambulatory blood pressure for the two sub-groups and for all

422 patients. In each instance, the average AOBP reading was similar to the corresponding awake ambulatory blood pressure. These results were important from two perspectives. First, the data were collected from patients in the community and not in a research centre. Second, the results demonstrated that a separate examining room was not essential for obtaining an AOBP reading. One of the major criticisms of AOBP was no longer valid.

The results of SPRINT had been criticized because AOBP had been used to record the office blood pressure. Much of this criticism originated from a sub-study (76) of SPRINT that had reported an average AOBP (120/66) in the lower treatment target group that was less than their awake ambulatory blood pressure (127/72). This finding was unexpected, since comparisons between AOBP and awake ambulatory blood pressure at systolic readings above 130 mmHg were similar. The finding in SPRINT prompted me to examine other studies which had compared the awake ambulatory blood pressure with office blood pressure recorded using different measurement techniques when the average readings were less than 130 mmHg. It turned out that office BP in research studies was always lower than the awake ambulatory blood pressure, regardless of how the office readings were measured. AOBP, mercury sphygmomanometers and other automated recorders all gave the same results (84).

These observations had ramifications beyond SPRINT and AOBP. The new target for lowering BP (77, 85) with medication was a systolic reading of either less than 120 mmHg or 130 mmHg, depending on the patients' other health issues. The best predictor of cardiovascular risk in relation to an individual's blood pressure status was the ambulatory blood pressure. There seemed to be a tacit assumption that the office readings were also an accurate representation of the patient's blood pressure status. The available evidence indicated that this was not necessarily true. As of today, we still do not know the best technique for office blood pressure measurement below the treatment target for many patients. The lack of data is especially true for manual office blood pressure readings in routine clinical practice, since no studies have been done with this method of measurement. From a patient's perspective, it doesn't much matter if office blood pressure readings are a little higher or a little lower, provided that the overall reading is normal.

AOBP had also been criticized because its readings were seen to be more variable and less consistent than with ambulatory and home blood pressure. This criticism was inherently misleading. AOBP was never proposed as a replacement for the out-of-office readings, whose advantages over office blood pressure have been supported by solid scientific evidence. Moreover, no studies had specifically examined the variability of AOBP. It was now time to do so.

Once again, I took the opportunity to go back in time. In 2009, I had collected data on 300 patients referred for 24-hour ambulatory blood pressure monitoring, who also had seven days of readings taken at home and an AOBP. In collaboration with Dr. Kaczorowski, the variability and agreement for AOBP and home blood pressure were each compared with the gold standard, awake ambulatory blood pressure. The comparative variability and agreement between the two pairs of readings were evaluated using several different types of statistical analyses. Overall, the relationship between AOBP and awake ambulatory blood pressure was similar to that of home blood pressure and awake ambulatory blood pressure. Since home blood pressure was considered to be an alternative to ambulatory blood pressure as a measure of cardiovascular risk, we concluded that the AOBP was not subject to excessive variability (86). Thus, another criticism of AOBP was shown to be inappropriate. However, we didn't go as far as to say that AOBP was as useful as home BP in diagnosing hypertension. More cardiovascular outcome data are needed before making such a statement.

In SPRINT (76), about one-quarter of the subjects had AOBP readings, except that the nurse remained in the room. The readings were otherwise recorded very carefully, according to guidelines and without any conversation. An analysis done after SPRINT had been completed showed that the nurse-attended and -unattended AOBP readings produced similar results. This finding introduced the idea that patients did not need to be alone for an AOBP reading. Nobody gave any reason why having someone in the room would otherwise be an advantage. In fact, the contrary was likely true. In clinical practice, having a nurse or doctor in the room during the measurement of the blood pressure would provide an opportunity for conversation, which is known to increase blood pressure and is probably responsible for much of the white coat effect associated with office readings in routine clinical practice. The concept of an attended AOBP was especially promoted by critics of AOBP in Europe.

Together with several colleagues, I set about finding all of the studies which compared attended and unattended AOBP. There were only five in number, but included 3,657 subjects. Analysis of the data showed that the attended systolic blood pressure was on average 5.8 mmHg higher than the unattended readings (87). This difference was statistically significant and was similar to the difference which had been previously reported (79) between AOBP and readings obtained with a mercury sphygmomanometer in other research studies. Thus, a carefully done office blood pressure reading in a research study, whether manual or attended AOBP, was higher than a proper AOBP reading, which, as you may recall, was similar to the awake ambulatory and home blood pressures, the best predictors of future cardiovascular disease.

So, the arguments based on AOBP not being feasible were reduced to doctors not wanting to spend money to purchase an AOBP recording device and to not wanting to re-design the office so that patients could rest in a quiet place alone. My belief that AOBP would eventually prevail as the preferred method in doctors' offices everywhere remains intact.

For those persons who haven't had their blood pressure recorded for a while, they should now expect to be left alone for readings to be taken several times with an automated device. If their doctor happens to still use a stethoscope, perhaps they should mention the Hypertension Canada or American Heart Association guidelines for blood pressure measurement. In countries such as Canada and the United States, hypertension should no longer be diagnosed solely on the basis of blood pressure readings recorded in the office. AOBP may be the best method for screening for possible hypertension, but a definitive diagnosis should be confirmed by 24-hour ambulatory blood pressure monitoring, or, if not feasible, then by seven days of self-measured readings recorded at home. Using this approach, inappropriate treatment for white coat hypertension can be avoided. AOBP can also be used to monitor the response to drug therapy, but a follow-up 24-hour ambulatory recording or home BP should be done to confirm that readings have become normal.

THIRTY

My Fiftieth Year Class Reunion

In May of each year, the University of Toronto celebrates class reunions of its various faculties and colleges. May 2018 marked the fiftieth anniversary of the graduation of my class from medical school. As part of the weekend's events, a session was held on the Saturday morning for presentations by class members related to interesting aspects of their professional lives. Years ago, at a previous reunion, I had done a presentation on 24-hour ambulatory blood pressure monitoring, which had been well received. This time, I chose automated office blood pressure measurement as a topic. This subject would be of interest to a wide audience, since every class member knew something about blood pressure measurement, even if it only related to their own diagnosis of hypertension.

I spoke for 30 minutes to a very attentive audience. When I finished, I received an enthusiastic reception, with class members saying how much they had enjoyed my talk. I had waited 50 years for this moment. As I said at the beginning, nothing I had ever done in medical school had been noteworthy. In a small way, I had now achieved the recognition that had previously evaded me during my years in university. We had our class reception on the Monday with the president of the University in attendance. Classmates were still coming up to me to congratulate me on my research. It may have been a minor event when compared to the other presentations I had given, but it had a special meaning for me, and one I will always remember.

Afterword

By now, it should be evident why being able to recognize opportunities for studies was such an important aspect of my success in research. I also believe that being different from my peers helped me to see topics for studies which were not as obvious to others. Being different when I was younger also made it easier to survive in an environment which is often hostile to researchers. Only a few of my colleagues who began their academic careers doing clinical research in the mid-1970s were able to sustain their efforts for more than five years. Not everyone could withstand the stress of writing grant proposals every year or two, without knowing if they would be approved for funding. Equally uncertain was the likelihood that research projects would be completed successfully. A prerequisite for success in research is to remain optimistic, despite having to endure periodic setbacks. Clinical practice always lurked in the background and often became irresistible, if one failed to achieve success early in a research career.

One of the secrets to my own success in research was to seek out collaborators, especially colleagues who knew more than I did about specific aspects of the studies. For years I was the only researcher in the Division of Cardiology at Sunnybrook, making it necessary for me to encourage the other clinical cardiologists to assist in recruiting patients or helping with other aspects of my research projects. At times, I had to venture further afield, to other hospitals, universities, cities and even countries in order to find collaborators whose expertise was essential to the project I was working on. The message here is that one should not hesitate to seek out others who might possess knowledge or other skills which can increase the likelihood of success. This approach may also lead to other collaborations, such as the working relationship which developed by keeping Dr. Kaczorowski involved in the CAMBO trial.

Somehow, the skills which I learned in order to survive being different when I was younger, allowed me to see what others did not see, not only in my main area of interest, hypertension, but also in other aspects of cardio-vascular disease, including stroke. In many ways, the opportunities seemed unlimited, since I was blessed with strong support from my colleagues with plenty of opportunities to satisfy my curiosity, while also advancing, albeit in a small way, our knowledge of common medical conditions.

There may be several useful "take-home" points from my story. The most obvious is that being different in childhood may seem unpleasant at the time, but this may provide skills which facilitate success in later life, and not only in medicine. My childhood wasn't uniformly bad. Although I was different from most of my playmates, I still had opportunities which they lacked. It is important to recognize opportunities which can make your life both more interesting and rewarding.

Although involvement in medical research may be different today, the attributes required for a successful career have probably not changed very much. Aspiring researchers should carefully evaluate what they are told, keeping in mind that there should always be good evidence to support the accepted beliefs. It should not be too difficult for a curious mind to discover aspects of clinical practice which still require further studies to confirm their validity. As in the past, training at the best possible centres will enhance the likelihood of success in the future. Having helpful mentors and discovering colleagues whose knowledge complements your own will also make it easier to address important issues in need of further research. Perseverance is often required to be in a position to benefit from chance observations.

Finally, for readers who are still early in their careers, it is possible to achieve success later in life, by applying your experiences from the past to deal with challenges and opportunities you will encounter, not only in medicine but in other fields as well.

References

1. Dollery CT, Lewis PJ, Myers MG, Reid JL. Central hypotensive effect of propranolol in the rabbit. British Journal of Pharmacology 1973;48:343.
2. Reid JL, Lewis PJ, Myers MG, Dollery, CT. Cardiovascular effects of intracerebroventricular d-, l- and dl-propranolol in the conscious rabbit. Journal of Pharmacology and Experimental Therapeutics 1974;188:394–399.
3. Myers MG, Reid JL, Lewis PJ. The effect of central serotonin depletion of DOCA-saline hypertension in the rat. Cardiovascular Research 1974;8:806–814.
4. Myers MG, Lewis PJ, Reid JL, Dollery CT. Brain concentration of propranolol in relation to hypotensive effect in the rabbit with observations on brain propranolol levels in man. Journal of Pharmacology and Experimental Therapeutics 1975;192:327–335.
5. Myers MG, Lewis GRJ, Steiner J, Dollery CT. Clinical evaluation of atenolol in essential hypertension. Clinical Pharmacology and Therapeutics 1976;19:502–507.
6. Myers MG and Thiessen JJ. Pharmacokinetic and dose-response evaluation of metoprolol in hypertensive patients. Clinical Pharmacology and Therapeutics 1980;27:756–762.
7. Myers MG. Hydrochlorothiazide +/- amiloride in the treatment of hypertension in the elderly—a dose-titration study. Archives of Internal Medicine 1987;174:1026–1031.
8. Hulley SB, Furberg CD, Gurland B, McDonald R, Perry HM, Schnaper HW, et al. Systolic Hypertension in the Elderly Program (SHEP): Antihypertensive efficacy of chlorthalidone. American Journal of Cardiology 1985;56:913–920.
9. SHEP Cooperative Research Group. Prevention of stroke by antihypertensive drug treatment in older persons with isolated systolic hypertension: final results of the Systolic Hypertension in the Elderly Program (SHEP). Journal of the American Medical Association 1991;265:3255–3264.
10. Levene DL, Myers MG. Catheter-induced coronary spasm; Canadian Medical Association Journal 1974;111:647.

11. Myers MG, Arshinoff SA. Infection and pheochromocytoma. Journal of the American Medical Association 1977;237:2095.

12. Myers MG, Shulman HS, Saibil EA, Naqvi SZ. Variation in measurement of coronary lesions on 35 and 70 mm angiograms. American Journal of Roentgenology 1978;130:913–916.

13. Kannel WB. Blood pressure and the development of cardiovascular disease in the aged, in Cardiology in Old Age. Plenum Publishers, New York, 1976, p 143.

14. Myers MG, Kearns PM, Kennedy DS, Fisher RH. Postural hypotension and diuretic therapy in the elderly. Canadian Medical Association Journal 1978;199:581–585.

15. Myers MG, Weingert ME, Fisher RH, Gryce CI, Shulman HS. Unnecessary diuretic therapy in the elderly. Age and Ageing 1982;11:213–21.

16. Myers MG, Kearns PM, Shedletsky R, Lysak AA, Fisher RH. Postural hypotension and mental function in the elderly. Canadian Medical Association Journal 1978;119:1065.

17. Myers MG, Iazzetta JJ. Effect of topical intranasal phenylephrine on blood pressure. Canadian Medical Association Journal 1982;127:365–368.

18. Myers MG. Beta-adrenoceptor antagonism and the pressor response to phenylephrine. Clinical Pharmacology and Therapeutics 1984;36:57–63.

19. Miller RR, Olson HJ, Amsterdam EA, Mason DT. Propranolol withdrawal rebound phenomenon. New England Journal of Medicine 1975;293:416–418.

20. Myers MG, Wisenberg G. Sudden withdrawal of propranolol in patients with angina pectoris. Chest 1977;71:24–26.

21. Myers MG, Freeman MR, Wisenberg G, Juma Z. Propranolol withdrawal in patients with angina pectoris - a prospective study. American Heart Journal 1979;97:298–303.

22. Olivieri NF, Brittenham GM, McLaren CE, Templeton, Cameron RG, McClelland RA, et al. Long-term safety and effectiveness of iron-chelation therapy with deferiprone for thalassemia major. New England Journal of Medicine 1998;339:417–423.

23. Norris JW, Hachinski VC, Myers MG, Callow J, Wong T, Moore RW. Serum cardiac enzymes in stroke. Stroke 1979;10:548–553.

24. Myers MG, Norris JW, Hachinski VC, Sole MJ. Plasma norepinephrine in stroke. Stroke 1981;12:200–204.

25. Myers MG, Leenen FHH, Burns R, Frankel D. Nifedipine tablet vs hydralazine in patients with persisting hypertension who receive combined diuretic and beta-blocker therapy. Clinical Pharmacology and Therapeutics 1986;39:409–413.

26. Myers MG, Raemsch KD. Comparative pharmacokinetics and antihypertensive effects of the nifedipine tablet and capsule. Journal of Cardiovascular Pharmacology 1987;10 (supplement X):S76-8.

27. Myers MG, Baigrie RS, Dubbin JD. Nifedipine versus propranolol treatment of unstable angina in the elderly. Canadian Journal of Cardiology 1988;4:402–6.

28. Psaty BM, Heclbert SR, Koepsell TD, et al. The risk of myocardial infarction associated with antihypertensive therapy. Journal of the American Medical Association 1995;274;620–625.

29. Furberg CD, Psaty BM, Meyer JV. Nifedipine. Dose-related mortality in patients with coronary heart disease. Circulation 1995;92:1326–1331.

30. Myers MG, Carruthers SG, Leenen FHH, Haynes RB. Canadian Hypertension Society Consensus Conference on the Pharmacologic Treatment of Hypertension. Canadian Medical Association Journal 1989;140:1141–6.

31. Myers MG. "Drug may have caused huge number of deaths": lessons learned during an encounter with The Fifth Estate. Canadian Medical Association Journal 1996; 155:772–775.

32. Carruthers SG. Calcium channel blocker on trial: hypertension specialists win landmark libel suit against Canadian Broadcasting Corporation. Journal of Hypertension 2002;20:1663–1666.

33. Myers MG, Cairns JA, Singer J. The consent form as a possible cause of side-effects. Clinical Pharmacolology and Therapeutics 1987;42:2503.

34. Cairns JA, Gent M, Singer J, Finnie KJ, Froggatt GM, Holder DA, et al. (incl. Myers MG). Aspirin sulfinpyrazone or both in unstable angina. New England Journal of Medicine 1985;313:1369–75.

35. Lewis HD Jr, Davis JW, Archibald GD, et al. Protective effect of aspirin against acute myocardial infarction and death in men with unstable angina. New England Journal of Medicine 1983;309:396–403.

36. Sutherland DJ, McPherson DD, Renton KW, Spencer A, Montague T. The effect of caffeine on rate, rhythm and ventricular repolarization. Chest 1985; 87:319–324.

37. Myers MG, Harris L, Leenen FHH, Grant D. Caffeine as a possible cause of ventricular arrhythmias. American Journal of Cardiology 1987;59:1024–8.

38. Myers MG, Harris L. High dose caffeine and ventricular arrhythmias. Canadian Journal of Cardiology 1990;6:95–98.

39. Colton T, Gosselin RE, Smith RP. The tolerance of coffee drinkers to caffeine. Clinical Pharmacology and Therapeutics 1968;9:31–39.

40. Myers MG. Caffeine and cardiac arrhythmias. Annals of Internal Medicine 1991;114:147–50.

41. Myers MG, Basinski A. Coffee and coronary heart disease. Archives of Internal Medicine 1992;152:1767–72.

42. Myers MG. Effects of caffeine on blood pressure. Archives of Internal Medicine 1988;148:1189–93.

43. Myers MG, Reeves RA. Caffeine and ambulatory blood pressure. American Journal of Hypertension 1993;6:91–6.

44. Myers MG, Benowitz NL, Dubbin JD, Haynes RB, Sole MJ. The cardiovascular effects of smoking in patients with ischemic heart disease. Chest 1988;93:14–19.

45. Myers MG, Baigrie RS, Charlat ML, Morgan CD. Are routine non-invasive tests useful in predicting outcome post-myocardial infarction in the elderly? Lancet 1993;342:1069–73.

46. Coats AJS, Adamopoulos S, Meyer TE, Conway J, Sleight P. Effects of physical training in chronic heart failure. Lancet 1990;335:63–66.

47. Kavanaugh T, Myers MG, Baigrie RS, Mertens DJ, Sawyer P, Sheppard RJ. Quality of life and cardiorespiratory function in chronic heart failure: effects of 12 months' aerobic training. Heart 1996;76:42–49.

48. Myers MG. Self-measurement of blood pressure at home—the potential for reporting bias. Blood Pressure Monitoring 1998;3(suppl 1):S19–S22.

49. Mengden T, Hernandez Medina RM, Beltran B, Alvarez E, Kraft K, Vetter H. Reliability of reporting self-measurement of blood pressure values by hypertensive patients. American Journal of Hypertens 1998;11:1413–1417.

50. Myers MG, Stergiou GS. Reporting bias: The Achilles heel of home blood pressure measurement. Journal of the American Society of Hypertension 2014;8:350–357.

51. Editorial. Standardization of methods of measuring the arterial blood pressure. British Heart Journal 1939;1:261–267.

52. Myers MG, Reeves RA. White coat phenomenon in patients receiving antihypertensive therapy. American Journal of Hypertension 1991;4:844–9.

53. Myers MG, Oh P, Reeves RA, Joyner CD. Prevalence of white coat effect in the community. American Journal of Hypertension 1995;8:591–597.

54. Myers MG, Reeves RA. White coat effect in treated hypertensive patients - gender differences. Journal of Human Hypertension 1995;9:729–733.

55. Myers MG, Haynes RB, Rabkin SW. Canadian Hypertension Society guidelines for ambulatory blood pressure monitoring. American Journal of Hypertension 1999;12:1149–1157.

56. Myers MG, Meglis G, Polemidiotis G. The impact of physician versus automated blood pressure readings on office-induced hypertension. Journal of Human Hypertension 1997;11:491–493.

57. Myers MG, Valdivieso M. Use of an automated blood pressure recording device, the BpTRU, to reduce the "white coat effect" in routine practice. American Journal of Hypertension 2003;16:494–497.

58. Beckett L, Godwin M. The BpTRU automatic blood pressure monitor compared to 24-h ambulatory blood pressure monitoring in the assessment of blood pressure in patients with hypertension. BMC Cardiovascular Disorders 2005;5:18.

59. Leenen FHH, Dumais J, McInnis N, Turton P, Stratychuk L, Nemeth K, et al: 2006 Ontario survey on the prevalence and control of hypertension (ON BP). Canadian Medical Association Journal 2008;178:1441–9.

60. Myers MG, Godwin M, Dawes M, Kiss A, Tobe SW, Grant FC, Kaczorowski J. Conventional versus automated measurement of blood pressure in primary care patients with systolic hypertension: randomized, parallel design, controlled trial. British Medical Journal. 2011;342:d286.

61. Myers MG, Godwin M, Dawes M, Kiss A, Tobe SW, Kaczorowski J. Conventional versus automated measurement of blood pressure in the office (CAMBO) trial. Family Practice 2012;29:376–382.

62. Myers MG: Automated blood pressure measurement in routine clinical practice. Blood Pressure Monitoring 2006;11:59–62.

63. Myers MG, Valdivieso M, Kiss A. Optimum frequency of office blood pressure measurement using an automated sphygmomanometer. Blood Pressure Monitoring 2008; 13:333–338.

64. Myers MG, Valdivieso M, Kiss A. Consistent relationship with automated office blood pressure recorded in different settings. Blood Pressure Monitoring 2009;14:108–111.

65. Myers MG, Valdivieso M, Kiss A. Use of automated office blood pressure measurement to reduce the white coat response. Journal of Hypertension 2009;27:280–286.

66. Myers MG, Valdivieso M, Chessman M, Kiss A. Can sphygmomanometers designed for self-management of blood pressure in the home be used in office practice? Blood Pressure Monitoring 2010;13:300–304.

67. Myers MG, Kaczorowski J. Office blood pressure is lower than awake ambulatory blood pressure at lower targets for treatment. Journal of Clinical Hypertension 2017;19:1210–1213.

68. Myers MG, Valdivieso M. Evaluation of an automated sphygmomanometer for use in the office setting. Blood Pressure Monitoring 2012;17:116–119.

69. Rabi DM, Daskalopoulou SS, Padwal RS, Khan NA, Grover SA, Hackam DG, et al. The 2011 Canadian Hypertension Education Program Recommendations for the Management, Diagnosis, Assessment of Risk, and Therapy. Canadian Journal of Cardiology 2011;27:415–433.

70. Kaczorowski J, Chambers LW, Dolovich L, Paterson MJ, Karwalajtys T, Gierman T, et al. Improving cardiovascular health at the population level: 39 community cluster randomized trial of Cardiovascular Health Awareness Program (CHAP). British Medical Journal 2011;342:d442.

71. Myers MG, Kaczorowski J, Paterson M, Dolovich L, Tu, K. Thresholds for diagnosing hypertension based upon cardiovascular outcomes using automated office blood pressure. Hypertension 2015; 66:489–495.

72. Myers MG, Kaczorowski J, Dolovich L, Tu K, Paterson JM. Cardiovascular risk in hypertension in relation to achieved blood pressure using automated office blood pressure measurement. Hypertension 2016;68:866–872

73. Leung AA, Nerenberg . Daskalopoulou SS, McBrien K, Zarnke KB, Dasgupta K et al. Hypertension Canada's 2016 CHEP Guidelines for Blood Pressure Measurement, Diagnosis, Assessment of Risk, Prevention and Treatment of Hypertension. Canadian Journal of Cardiology 2016;32:569–588.

74. Kaczorowski J, Myers MG, Gelfer M, Dawes M, Mang EJ, Berg A, et al. D. How do family physicians measure blood pressure in routine clinical practice? Canadian Family Physician 2017;63:e193–199.

75. The SPRINT Research Group. A randomized trial of intensive versus standard blood pressure control. New England Journal of Medicine 2015;373:2103–2116.

76. Johnson KC, Whelton PK, Cushman WC, Cutler JA, Evans GW, Snyder JK, et al. for the SPRINT Research Group. Blood pressure measurement in SPRINT (Systolic Blood Pressure Intervention Trial). Hypertension 2018;71:848–857.

77. Whelton PK, Carey RM, Aronow WS, Casey DE, Collins CJ, Himmelfarb CD, et al. 2017 ACC/AHA/AAPA/ABC/ACPM/AGS/APhA/ASH/ASPC/NMA/PCNA guideline for the prevention, detection, evaluation, and management of high blood Pressure in adults: a report of the American College of Cardiology/American Heart Association Task Force on Clinical Practice Guidelines. Hypertension. 2018;71:1269–1324.

78. Pickering TG, Hall JE, Appel LJ, Falkner BE, Graves J, Hill MN, et al. Recommendations for blood pressure measurement in humans and experimental animals Part 1: blood pressure measurement in humans a statement for professionals from the subcommittee of Professional and Public Education of the Am Heart Association Council on High Blood Pressure Research. Hypertension 2005;45:142–161.

79. Roerecke M, Kaczorowski J, Myers MG. Comparing automated office blood pressure readings with other methods of blood pressure measurement for identifying patients with possible hypertension. A systematic review and meta-analysis. Journal of the American Medical Association—Internal Medicine 2019;179:351–362.

80. Muntner P, Shimbo D, Carey RM, Charleston JB, Gaillard T, Misra S, et al. Measurement of blood pressure in humans. A scientific statement from the American Heart Association. Hypertension 2019;73:e35–e66.

81. Williams B, Mancia G, Spiering W, Agatibi Rosei E, Azizi M, Burnier M, et al. 2018 ESC/ESH guidelines for the management of arterial hypertension. Journal of Hypertension 2018;36:1953–2041.

82. Mancia G, Fagard R, Krzysztof N, Redon J, Zanchetti A, Bohm M et al. 2013 ESH/ESC guidelines for the management of arterial hypertension. Journal of

Hypertension 2013; 31:1281–1357.

83. Armstrong D, Matangi M, Brouillard D, Myers MG. Automated office blood pressure—being alone and not location is what matters most. Blood Pressure Monitoring 2015;20:204–8.

84. Myers MG, Kaczorowski J. Office blood pressure is lower than awake ambulatory blood pressure at lower targets for treatment. Journal of Clinical Hypertension 2017;19:1210–1213.

85. Nerenberg KA, Zarnke KB, Leung AA, Dasgupta K, Butalia S, McBrien K, et al. Hypertension Canada's 2018 guidelines for diagnosis, risk assessment, prevention and treatment of hypertension in adults and children. Canadian Journal of Cardiology 2018;34:506–525.

86. Myers MG, Kaczorowski J. Are Automated Office Blood Pressure Readings More Variable than Home Readings? Hypertension 2020;75:1179–1183.

87. Myers MG, de La Sierra A, Roerecke M, Kaczorowski J. Attended versus unattended automated office blood pressure measurement in the diagnosis and treatment of Journal of Hypertension 2020;38:1407–1411.

Acknowledgement of Collaborators

John L. Reid, Department of Clinical Pharmacology, Hammersmith Hospital

Peter J. Lewis, Department of Clinical Pharmacology, Hammersmith Hospital

Colin T. Dollery, Department of Clinical Pharmacology, Hammersmith Hospital

Gerald R. J. Lewis, Department of Clinical Pharmacology, Hammersmith Hospital

Jan Steiner, Department of Clinical Pharmacology, Hammersmith Hospital

Jake J. Thiessen, Faculty of Pharmacy, University of Toronto

Donald L. Levene, Division of Cardiology, Sunnybrook Health Sciences Centre

Steven A. Arshinoff, Division of Cardiology, Sunnybrook Health Sciences Centre

Salim Z. Naqvi, Division of Cardiology, Sunnybrook Health Sciences Centre

Harry S. Shulman, Department of Radiology, Sunnybrook Health Sciences Centre

Eric A. Saibil, Department of Radiology, Sunnybrook Health Sciences Centre

Patricia M. Kearns. Department of Nursing, Sunnybrook Health Sciences Centre

Ralph Shedletsky, Department of Psychology, Sunnybrook Health Scinces Centre

Anthony A. Lysak, Department of Psychology, Sunnybrook Health Sciences Centre

Rory H. Fisher, Division of Geriatrics, Sunnybrook Health Sciences Centre

John J. Iazzetta, Department of Pharmacy, Sunnybrook Health Sciences Centre

Gerald Wisenberg, Division of Cardiology, Sunnybrook Health Sciences Centre

Michael R. Freeman, Division of Cardiology, Sunnybrook Health Sciences Centre

Zulfikar Juma, Division of Cardiology, Sunnybrook Health Sciences Centre

John W. Norris, Division of Neurology, Sunnybrook Health Sciences Centre

Vladimir C. Hachinski, Division of Neurology, Sunnybrook Health Sciences Centre

John Callow, Department of Pharmacology, University of Toronto

Robert W. Moore, Department of Biochemistry, Sunnybrook Health Sciences Centre

Michel J. Sole, Division of Cardiology, Toronto General Hospital

Frans H. H. Leenen, Division of Clinical Pharmacology, Toronto Western Hospital

David Frankel, Miles Laboratories, Toronto

Klaus D. Raemsch, Bayer Inc. Leverkusen, West Germany

James D. Dubbin, Division of Cardiology, Sunnybrook Health Sciences Centre

S. George Carruthers, Division of Clinical Pharmacology, University of Western Ontario

R. Brian Haynes, Department of Clinical Epidemiology, McMaster University

John A. Cairns, Division of Cardiology, University of Western Ontario

Joel Singer, Department of Medicine, Toronto General Hospital

Louise Harris, Division of Cardiology, Sunnybrook Health Sciences Centre

Denis Grant, Department of Pharmacology, University of Toronto

Anthony Basinski, Institute of Clinical and Evaluative Sciences, Sunnybrook Health Sciences Centre

Richard A. Reeves, Division of Clinical Pharmacology, Sunnybrook Health Sciences Centre

Neil L. Benowitz, Division of Clinical Pharmacology, San Francisco General Hospital

Martin L. Charlat, Division of Cardiology, Sunnybrook Health Sciences Centre

Christopher D. Morgan, Division of Cardiology, Sunnybrook Health Sciences Centre

Terence Kavanagh, Cardiac Unit, Toronto Rehabilitation Centre

George S. Stergiou, Department of Medicine, University of Athens

Paul Oh, Division of Clinical Pharmacology, Sunnybrook Health Sciences Centre

Campbell D. Joyner, Division of Cardiology, Sunnybrook Health Sciences Centre

Simon W. Rabkin, Division of Cardiology, University of British Columbia

Gus Meglis, Department of Family Medicine, Sunnybrook Health Sciences Centre

George Polemidiotis, Department of Family Medicine, Sunnybrook Health Sciences Centre

Miguel Valdivieso, Division of Cardiology, Sunnybrook Health Sciences Centre

Marshall Godwin, Department of Family Medicine, Memorial University

Martin Dawes, Department of Family Medicine, McGill University

Alexander Kiss, Institute of Clinical and Evaluative Sciences, Sunnybrook Health Sciences Centre

Sheldon W. Tobe, Division of Nephrology, Sunnybrook Health Sciences Centre

Janusz Kaczorowski, Department of Family Medicine, University of British Columbia

F. Curry Grant, Department of Medicine, Belleville General hospital

Michael Paterson, Institute of Clinical and Evaluative Sciences, Sunnybrook Health Sciences Centre

Karen Tu, Institute of Clinical and Evaluative Sciences, Sunnybrook Health Sciences Centre

Lisa Dolovich, Department of Family Medicine, McMaster University

Michael Roerecke, Department of Psychiatry, Centre for Addiction and Mental Health

Murray Matangi, Kingston Heart Centre

Alejandro de la Sierra, Department of Internal Medicine, University of Barcelona

www.ingramcontent.com/pod-product-compliance
Lightning Source LLC
Chambersburg PA
CBHW051258020426
42333CB00026B/3260